DIABETES TYPE II
AND WHAT TO DO

OTHER BOOKS

by

June Biermann and Barbara Toohey:

The Peripatetic Diabetic
The Diabetes Question and Answer Book
The Diabetic's Sports and Exercise Book
The Diabetic's Book: All Your Questions Answered
The Diabetic Woman (with Lois Jovanovic-Peterson, M.D.)
The Diabetic Man (with Peter A. Lodewick, M.D.)
The Diabetic's Total Health Book
Psyching Out Diabetes (with Richard R. Rubin, Ph.D.)

Diabetes Type II

and What to Do

Virginia Valentine, R.N., M.S., C.D.E.,
June Biermann and Barbara Toohey

Lowell House
Los Angeles
Contemporary Books
Chicago

Valentine, Virginia.
    Diabetes type II and what to do / Virginia Valentine, June Biermann, and Barbara
Toohey.
        p.   cm.
    ISBN 1-56565-149-9
    1. Non-insulin-dependent diabetes—Popular works.   I. Biermann, June.   II. Toohey,
Barbara.   III. Title.   IV. Title: Diabetes, type 2 and you and what to do.
    RC660.4.V35   1993
    616.4'62—dc20   92-37694
                                                                                        CIP

Requests for such permissions should be addressed to:
Lowell House
2029 Century Park East, Suite 3290
Los Angeles, CA 90067

Publisher: Jack Artenstein
Vice-President/Editor-in-Chief: Janice Gallagher
Director of Publishing Services: Mary D. Aarons
Text design: Hespenheide Design

Manufactured in the United States of America
10 9 8 7 6 5 4 3 2 1

TABLE OF CONTENTS

I dedicate this book to my late mother, Myrna Valentine,
who was a Type II diabetic and the epitome of what every
nurse should be; to my daughter, Melanie, who will most likely
become a Type II diabetic and who I hope will grow up into a world
without diabetes; to the world's best husband, John McLaughlin; and
to my adopted sister, B. J. Christopher.
—VV

We dedicate this book with love and appreciation
to Dan Chilton, whose protean talents and Herculean efforts caused
the phoenix to rise from the ashes.
—JB & BT

FOREWORD

The philosopher Peter Nivio Zarlenga said, "It is hard to begin to move when you don't know where you are moving, how to move, or if you are going to get there."

The path to your future good health begins with finding out that you have Type II diabetes. This is the moment of realization that your future is truly in your hands. At that moment, knowing you are diabetic, you are no longer the victim of an unseen enemy. You can begin to make decisions that will determine which path your life and health will take.

June Biermann, Barbara Toohey, and Virginia Valentine do not, to paraphrase Shakespeare, "rail against a sea of troubles, but indeed take arms against it and in so doing resist it." Type II diabetes mellitus, more than any other disease known to mankind, is "resistible." The patient with this disease is not doomed. Our knowledge as to the cause and nature of this disease has increased exponentially, and in Type II diabetes mellitus knowledge is truly power. June, Barbara, and Virginia have given people with this infirmity the power to control their disease and influence their future. We have traveled a long path in a short time from the vision that things just happen at random to people with diabetes mellitus. Along the path, we have gained the understanding and the actions necessary to effect changes. As health-care professionals we have learned that Type II diabetes mellitus demands to be taken as seriously as Type I and that the patient plays the most important part in the preservation of good health.

One cannot construct something of worth without quality tools and raw materials, just as one cannot embark on a path without a guide who is up-to-date, accurate, and above all useful. The tools necessary to create the state we call good health are all presented by June and Barbara in their unique, straightforward, and always understandable and enjoyable style. What is found in this book will empower and serve as a road map to readers and enable them to take an active, enlightened, and vital role in the most important job they have ever had to assume to survive—helping themselves and helping others to guarantee the success of the treatment of a disease that above all else is treatable.

With this book we are not only given a road map, however, but also our own personal guide: Virginia Valentine. Like an experienced explorer who has been on a voyage of exploration, Virginia Valentine has come back home to help lead us all to the promised land. Rather than leading us at arms length, as is all too often the way health professionals teach their patients, Virginia Valentine shares with us her own personal successes and failures, what caused them, and the results that ensued. She literally puts her arm around the reader and opens not only her mind but also her heart to her disciples and students both new and old.

As one of the multitude who has watched the role of patients with Type II diabetes mellitus change from being the object of orders and the receptacle of instructions to the current and only acceptable role, that of equal partners in their health care, I am happy to be able to express from all of us to June Biermann, Barbara Toohey, and Virginia Valentine our heart-felt thanks for their book and their efforts, which have helped evoke this change in attitude and knowledge, and most important, for continuing to teach us and keep us on the right path.

Alan O. Marcus, M.D., F.A.C.P.
South Orange County Endocrinology
Mission Viejo, California

THE BEST KIND OF DIABETES YOU CAN HAVE

June Biermann and Barbara Toohey

Several years ago a dermatologist removed a small growth near Barbara's left eye. The lab report came back indicating it had been malignant. The doctor was very reassuring. "It's all taken care of. You don't have to worry or even think about it. Just always wear a sunscreen when you're outdoors. It's the best kind of cancer you can have."

Many people who are diagnosed as having diabetes in their adult years are told something similar: "You have borderline diabetes," or "You have mild diabetes," or "You have a touch of diabetes; just stay away from sugar and lose some weight and you'll be fine." If the words, "It's the best kind of diabetes you can have" aren't actually spoken, the implication is there. And if it isn't there, you come up with it yourself. When June was diagnosed at age 45, she was disturbed and upset, of course, but kept saying to herself—and to anyone else who would listen—"At least I don't have the kind of diabetes that you have to take insulin for, so it's not so bad."

Later on when it turned out that she did have to take insulin after all, she immediately felt that her kind of diabetes was much more serious and that those who didn't have to take insulin really had it easy. She's ashamed to admit that once when she was feeling particularly frustrated and resentful over her own problems with diabetes, she bitterly referred to those who can get along on diet and exercise (or diet and exercise and pills) as "those fake diabetics." Her attitude was, "All they need to do is lose some weight. That's not hard to do." (This from a person who has been skinny all her life, has no taste for sweets, and isn't even all that much interested in food.)

But the more we learned about "the other diabetes" as author Doro Sims, who has diabetes herself, calls it, the more we learned that the grass is definitely not greener on one side of the diabetes fence or the other. Both sides have an equal share of weeds and bare spots, gopher holes and snakes in the grass. We assure you that we're totally reformed now and we take all manifestations of diabetes equally seriously.

Unfortunately not everyone who has diabetes takes the condition so seriously. Whether their attitude has been fostered by reassuring doctors or self-created as a defense mechanism, the vast majority of people who develop diabetes as adults feel "it's not that big a deal" and go on to act accordingly: testing their blood sugars seldom or never, maybe exercising and maybe not, maybe changing their eating patterns and maybe not.

The more we saw this casual and lackadaisical approach to diabetes in action and the more we saw the health problems and diabetes complications that resulted from it, the more we realized that Something Had to Be Done. We wanted to alert this vast majority of diabetics to the fact that it is as important for them to handle their disease with serious care and attention as it is for those who have been shooting up insulin since childhood.

Because we have such great respect for diabetic endocrinologist Lois Jovanovic-Peterson, M.D., with whom we collaborated on *The Diabetic Woman,* we wrote to her half-jokingly: "How would you like to put on 30 pounds and stop taking insulin? The reason we ask is that we really think there needs to be a book on adult diabetes. Janice, our editor, thinks so, too, because her mother just developed it and Janice is struggling trying to help her make the necessary changes in her life. We figured that if you wrote this book with us, it would give it that extra push of authority if you had Type II diabetes [the most typical kind for people diagnosed in their middle or later years]."

Dr. Jovanovic-Peterson was quick to respond that she agreed such a book needed to be written, and that it would be a thousand times more meaningful if our collaborator had Type II diabetes. For that reason she suggested someone other than herself. Her recommendation was a person whom she described as "a Type II who uses her condition to motivate and win the hearts and minds of other Type II's. She has won the "Educator of the Year" award for the state of Oklahoma and the national award from the American Association of Diabetes Educators. She is witty, clever, and smart, too." She was referring to Virginia Valentine, R.N., C.D.E., Clinical Nurse Specialist for diabetes at the University of New Mexico Medical Center in Albuquerque, New Mexico, and Diabetes Educator of the Presbyterian Diabetes Center in Albuquerque, New Mexico. She is also Clinical Associate faculty at the University of New Mexico College of Nursing.

Everything Dr. Jovanovic-Peterson said about Virginia proved to be true—and then some!—as we quickly learned and as you will see in this book.

We will now put our three heads and two somewhat impaired pancreases together to help you develop an adult attitude toward your adult-onset diabetes, an attitude that will make it possible for you to make sure that your diabetes truly is the best kind of diabetes you can have—the well-controlled kind!

I Don't Have A Character Flaw—And Neither Do You!

Virginia Valentine, R.N., M.S., C.D.E.

I have had Type II diabetes for 12 years. I was diagnosed at age 31, which, as most textbooks will tell you, is much too young to get this type of diabetes. In the recent past, many times when I introduced myself to an audience, I would share with them the fact that I had Type II diabetes, but I always made sure to let them know that I was not yet 40. Too bad I can no longer use that disclaimer.

Most people, when they're diagnosed with diabetes, ask, "Why me, Lord?" But since there was so much history of diabetes on both sides of my family, I guess I always knew that eventually I would get it. My question was, "Why *now,* Lord? I wasn't supposed to get diabetes until after the age of 40. Although I felt a little cheated at getting it at such an early age, I wasn't all that worried because my paternal grandfather, who had diabetes, lived to be almost 80, and my mother's diabetic aunts and cousins didn't have any of the terrible complications that I was to see later when I went to work in the field of diabetes.

I chose to go into nursing after several years in college as an art and advertising major when I realized that I wanted to do something that had a more significant impact on people. My mother was a nurse, but I had not previously considered nursing because I thought all nurses had to be as smart as she was—and I felt that let me out.

Then one summer after my sophomore year in college, I didn't have a summer job. You know how mothers can't stand it if they see you sleeping late and frittering away your time, so my mom made me come to the hospital to help out in the nursery. I was petrified of handling those little babies, but that summer I did discover two things that I'd not previously known or appreciated: (1) Most nurses were not as smart as my mom (which is not a put-down for nurses but praise for my mom, who was a genius), therefore I could probably handle the schooling; and (2) the essence of nursing is not shots and bedpans, but bringing out the inner healing reserves of people. That was the part of the job I really liked. I decided I would take college algebra and chemistry as a personal test to see if I could survive. I figured if I could live through those courses, I'd be able to manage nursing school. I could and I did.

In nursing school I discovered for myself something my mother had already told me: medical patients are much more interesting than surgical patients. Medical service is where they put the older patients with chronic diseases. Among health professionals the job of caring for patients with chronic diseases is not considered as glamorous as surgery, but I found the work much more rewarding and much more exciting. In medical service you get to know your patients and develop meaningful relationships with them.

A few years after graduating with a baccalaureate degree in nursing from Central State University in Oklahoma, I became pregnant with my first (and last!) baby. They told me I had gestational diabetes—that's the kind of diabetes that sometimes emerges during a pregnancy and then goes away after the baby is delivered. In 1976 most centers were not screening for gestational diabetes on a routine basis, but I was under the care of the university faculty, and they were checking for this. Although they recognized what it was, they didn't know much about treating it. Mainly what they did was to tell me to watch my sugar intake. (Sound familiar?) I followed their limited instructions except I didn't eat as many calories as they suggested. And still I had a 12-pound baby at full term. (In the past overweight babies were typical for women with diabetes.) She was beautiful, 25 inches long, with thick, dark, curly hair. She made all the other babies in the nursery look anemic.

Then, just as the textbooks tell you, five years later I was diagnosed with diabetes. At the time I was in graduate school at the University of Oklahoma College of Nursing specializing in chronic disease, and my husband and I were in the process of getting a divorce. (Could it be that I was under stress?) Since I was overweight and had very high blood sugar levels, my doctor immediately put me on insulin. I was on insulin for about a year before I decided to start figuring things out for myself. I lost 50 pounds and got off insulin and remained diet controlled for the next eight years. Three years ago I had to go onto oral hypoglycemic agents (pills) to control my blood sugar, and weight control is a never-ending battle for me.

In 1982 when I attended a diabetes management training program in New York with Dr. Lois Jovanovic-Peterson, I learned that women with diabetes didn't have to have 12-pound babies. To my sorrow, I also learned that my child would be at greatly increased risk for Type II diabetes herself, not only because I had Type II diabetes, but because she had developed increased fat cells during gestation. (I think motherhood should be renamed guilthood.)

Melanie is now 16 years old and overweight. It's something we have tried hard to avoid. We have watched the sugar and fat in the house, but she has always had a big appetite, and year after year I see her gain weight and struggle to deal with the excess weight and the social problems it brings. I hope this book will be useful to her when and if she does develop Type II diabetes and, before that, at the time she is having children, when she will likely have gestational diabetes. (Fortunately, this is a long way off because I have told her she can't have sex until she is 38 years old.)

Since 1981 I've primarily worked in areas helping people with diabetes. I love helping people with chronic diseases because they're so downtrodden—the stepchildren of the health care system. It's pretty amazing that people with diabetes are treated this way when you think about it, since diabetes affects 6 to 10 percent of the population in America. I consider it a privilege to be able to make a difference for people who have my affliction. I now work as a Clinical Nurse Specialist for the University of New Mexico

Medical Center in Albuquerque, which I consider the ideal job for me. I work with a superb team of health professionals who provide excellent diabetes care and are involved in leading edge research in diabetes. I guess the reason I enjoy working with folks with diabetes so much is that I see the health care system and society in general treat them as if they don't have a real disease. Many people—and that includes many health professionals who should know better—treat Type II diabetes as if it is only the punishment for being fat. The implication is that if you weren't fat you wouldn't have the disease and, therefore, it's all your own fault. I know this is true, because I've had more than one physician tell me the same.

That's why my message in this book is this: **Diabetes is not a character flaw!** If you believe that you have diabetes because you're fat, ask yourself these questions: Why are there so many people out there fatter than you who don't have diabetes? Why do half of the members of the Pima tribe of Native Americans in Arizona have Type II diabetes? Why do people with diabetes have parents and grandparents who also have diabetes?

I'll answer these questions for you. Type II diabetes in overweight people is a disorder in the way food is metabolized (converted to energy) and used in the body. Yes, lifestyle can affect diabetes, but when you look at the research reports on Type II, you see that the origin is in the genes you're born with. It is genetically determined, just like the color of your eyes. (And nobody calls your blue or brown eyes a character flaw!)

Probably in the next 10 years we'll see treatments directed toward the correction of these metabolic errors. What we have to do in the meantime is learn to live with the disease in such a way that we can stay healthy and participate fully in our lives. For me, participating fully in life means helping my patients and living in the mountains outside Albuquerque with the world's greatest husband and daughter. To do that I have to constantly work at diabetes management myself. The major challenge for me is to stay on a healthy diet and get some exercise every day.

The American Diabetes Association has as its mission "a world without diabetes." When I first saw that statement I tried to picture a world without diabetes and I couldn't stretch my imagination to visualize such a thing. Maybe the end of Type I diabetes can be achieved, but I can't bring myself to even dream of a world without Type II. I have to alter that phrase into "a world without *suffering* from diabetes." For me that means helping people keep their blood sugar in the near-normal range so they don't suffer the terrible, disabling complications of diabetes. It also means helping people make the necessary lifestyle changes for diabetes management without suffering—giving them commonsense approaches tailored to the individual. Above all, I want to keep them from feeling blamed for the disease they inherited.

For me, a world without suffering from diabetes is available right now, not something we have to wait for until a far-distant day. My reason for writing this book is to show you how together we can achieve this new kind of world for people with Type II diabetes.

TYPE II DIABETES: THE WHAT, WHO, AND WHY OF IT

June describes a scientific definition as "a term you don't understand explained in words you don't understand." Nowhere is this more true than in diabetes. When you're first diagnosed and have no idea of what diabetes is and how it's going to affect your life, wham!, you're hit with a whole bunch of scientific terms for your type of diabetes: Is it Type I? Type II? IDDM? NIDDM? Juvenile diabetes? Maturity-onset diabetes? Or several of the above?

We'll now explain these terms in words that you— and we!—can understand.

Type I is also called **juvenile diabetes** because it usually appears in childhood, adolescence, or sometimes early adulthood. Since in this type of diabetes the pancreas doesn't produce insulin, you have to take exogenous insulin. (Oops, we slipped in another scientific word on you. Exogenous insulin just means insulin produced outside your body that you inject.) For this reason it is also called **IDDM,** which stands for insulin-dependent diabetes mellitus. Most Type I's are of normal weight or even underweight.

Type II is also called **maturity-onset diabetes** because it usually appears in midlife or beyond. Often in this kind of diabetes the pancreas still produces insulin—maybe a lot of it—and you don't have to inject insulin. Because of this, it is also called **NIDDM,** meaning non-insulin-dependent diabetes mellitus. Most Type II's are overweight.

All this sounds pretty simple and cut-and-dried and easy to understand, doesn't it? Would that it were so—especially when it comes to people who are diagnosed as adults with Type II. When people are diagnosed diabetic in their middle or later years, they start reading up on the subject and find the advice to lose weight because that will help them keep their blood sugars normal. If they control their weight, they can probably get by on diet and exercise, or maybe diet and exercise and pills, and they won't have to inject insulin. We know this is true, because we've often said that about Type II's in our books.

But over the years, we've received numerous letters from people with diabetes who say, "I'm already underweight and they're telling me to lose more? I don't get it." (Ironically, June herself fits into this group.) Then there are those who are Type II (some overweight and some not) who wind up taking insulin to control their diabetes and they don't understand why since Type II's are supposed to have non-insulin-dependent diabetes. (That's June again!)

When we first met Virginia Valentine face-to-face at an American Association of Diabetes Educators' conference in Baltimore and began discussing the content of our mutual book, we posed the above conundrums to her. Her response was so quick and sure and logical that we knew she'd been thinking about and working through this problem herself.

Virginia divides people with Type II, maturity-onset diabetes into two subcategories: those who are insulin deficient and those who are insulin resistant. June is one of the former; Virginia is one of the latter. For convenience, we're going to refer to the two subcategories as Type II-D (deficient) and Type II-R (resistant).

Naturally, your major question now must be, "Where do I fit into these categories?" In this chapter, we'll ask

Virginia to help you figure out where you are so you'll
be able to find out in what direction you should go with
your diabetes therapy.

—June and Barbara

What You'll Find in This Chapter

Definitions of Diabetes
Type II-R (Resistant) and Type II-D (Deficient)
Diabetic Genes
"Thrifty" Genes
Who Gets Diabetes
Hypertension and Diabetes (Syndrome X)

JUNE AND BARBARA: Before we get into those Type II-R and D
categories, let's start out talking a little about diabetes in general.
As most of you already know, diabetes is a physical problem that
causes you to have too much sugar (glucose) in your blood. The
medical term for high blood sugar is hyperglycemia (*hyper* means
too much, and *glycemia* refers to glucose in the blood). This book
is all about how to turn hyperglycemia into euglycemia. That's the
term for a normal (not too low and not too high) level of sugar in
the blood. The word euglycemia has the same opening, *eu,* as in
euphoria, a feeling of happiness and well-being. And euphoria is
exactly what you'll feel when you get your hyperglycemia down to
euglycemia. The goal of all the advice and counsel in this book is
simply to move you into that ideal realm of normal blood sugar.

The American Diabetes Association defines diabetes as "a disease in which the body does not produce or respond to insulin (a
hormone produced by the pancreas). Without insulin, your body
cannot properly convert the food you eat into energy." They go on
to point out that diabetes is actually a general term for a number
of separate but related disorders. "These disorders fall into two
main categories: Type I and Type II."

Type I diabetes is a total lack of insulin caused by the fact that
the cells of the pancreas that normally produce insulin (beta cells)
have all been destroyed by the body's own immune system, which
has been triggered by a virus to attack the beta cells. As we said
before, since people with Type I diabetes make no insulin of their

own, they are called insulin-dependent. To get their blood sugars down into the normal range, they must inject insulin to be able to use the food they eat.

Type II diabetes, often defined as non-insulin-dependent, is much more complex both in cause and treatment. That's why we're happy to have Virginia here with us to explain this tough question of what Type II diabetes is. Let's start with the majority (90 percent) of Type II's, the ones we're calling the Type II-R's: those who are overweight and who have insulin resistance.

VIRGINIA: Understanding how diabetes develops and affects your body is the key to understanding how to control it. There are three problems that lead to this Type II-R diabetes. We'll take them in one-two-three order, although they don't necessarily develop in such a clear-cut way.

1. Insulin resistance and
hyperinsulemia (too much insulin)
In Type II-R diabetes the insulin produced by your pancreas does not work as it should because over the years your body cells have become resistant to it. They don't accept it as they once did. (Scientists aren't yet sure why this happens.) The cells in your body have receptors which, if working properly, accept the insulin. This coupling triggers a chain of events that open the cells to accept glucose (the sugar your body uses as fuel). If muscle cells don't use the glucose, it will be stored as fat.

When your body notices that your insulin isn't working to move glucose into the cells, it gets busy and makes more insulin. You then develop what we call hyperinsulemia, or too much insulin in your blood. Insulin is a powerful fat-generating hormone. This extra insulin, then, causes you to store fat and to be very hungry. By eating more to satisfy your insulin-induced hunger, you add even more weight. The extra fat caused by too much insulin and too much eating further increases your insulin resistance. Putting the two together, you now have the initial insulin resistance caused by Type II diabetes plus the additional insulin resistance caused by being overweight—a vicious cycle if ever there was one!

2. Inadequate insulin production

Now we come to the second of the three problems that cause Type II-R diabetes. So far the story is that you started many, many years before with insulin resistance. This caused your body to make extra insulin to try to move the glucose into your cells so that your blood sugar would stay normal. You probably had a weight problem to begin with and gained more weight over the years because of the extra insulin. When, then, did you actually become diabetic? When your body could no longer make enough extra insulin to compensate for the resistance. Let me make it clear that you're not really deficient in insulin—you're making way over the normal amount—but what you make is not enough, considering your needs, to keep your blood sugar at the normal level, so you end up with high blood sugar. In other words, you have diabetes.

3. Excess liver metabolism

Now you're insulin-resistant, without enough insulin even though you're still making a whole bunch of it, and your blood sugar is higher in the morning than it was when you went to bed. The explanation for this is that you have developed what we call excess liver glucose production. That's right, just when you thought things couldn't get worse, your liver gets into the act. When you haven't eaten in quite a few hours (since supper), your liver thinks it needs to start giving back some of the glucose it has stored up for this kind of an emergency. The liver either releases stored glucose or it can convert protein into glucose. When your liver starts kicking in after a six- or eight-hour fast, because your insulin resistance keeps the glucose from getting into the cells, the liver pours in extra glucose so you wake up with a terribly high blood sugar, even though it was normal when you went to bed.

To sum up, you have a resistance to insulin so your cells can't make use of insulin as they should. Your pancreas is making a lot of insulin but it's still not enough to overcome your resistance. And your liver doesn't understand why the glucose it's releasing isn't getting into your cells, so it does the only thing it knows how to do: it keeps producing more and more glucose, and that makes your blood sugar go higher and higher. That's how diabetes develops and keeps getting worse until you get proper treatment to bring it under control.

JUNE AND BARBARA: To help us understand all this better, could you tell us a typical story of how one individual's Type II-R diabetes might have developed over the years? Then each of our readers can visualize what probably happened to bring on his or her diabetes.

VIRGINIA: Yes, I can easily trace for you the physiological history of a typical case of Type II-R diabetes. Let's call the heroine of our story Helen. We'll say that she's 55 years old, overweight, feeling sluggish, has dry, itchy skin subject to frequent slow-healing infections and has tingling in her toes. She makes a doctor's appointment, is examined and tested, and is diagnosed with Type II diabetes. (These are typical symptoms, but sometimes there are absolutely no signs that would cue the person to go to the doctor.)

Helen's Story

Let's go back 10 to 20 years ago, when Helen develops the problem of insulin resistance (she is not aware of this, of course). To overcome this resistance her body starts making extra insulin to try to get the glucose from her food into the cells where it can be used as fuel. The extra insulin does keep her blood sugars normal, and therefore she is still nondiabetic. The extra insulin also causes her to gain weight, because it makes her store as fat a higher percentage of the food she eats. Soon she'll refer to herself as the type of person who can gain 5 pounds just smelling a plate of brownies—and she almost can!

After a few years, the excessive insulin she is making to compensate for her resistance is no longer enough. Now her pancreas starts losing its ability to produce the huge amounts of insulin she needs. My friend, Dr. Lois Jovanovic-Peterson, calls this "pancreatic poop-out." Normally when a person starts eating a meal, the body sends out a little squirt of insulin within minutes. This is called the first-phase insulin response. You can control your blood sugar a lot better if you have insulin right there at the door to meet the food than if you have to conquer a high blood sugar after the meal. Helen's body now refuses to send out enough insulin to cover that first-phase insulin response.

Look at the diagrams in Figure 1.1. The first shows how the normal pancreas sends out a small amount of insulin at the beginning of a meal, followed by a second-phase response that sends out a larger amount of insulin to keep the blood sugar from going up after the finish of the meal. The second bump of insulin prevents blood sugar from going up more than 20 or 40 points*. In other words, the person without diabetes who starts out with a blood sugar before meals of 70 or 80 may go up after the meal to 110 or 120. It's not normal to have wide swings in blood sugars throughout the day.

The second diagram shows what happens to blood sugar levels when you lose the first-phase insulin response. The blood sugar spikes up way above normal levels until the second phase kicks in.

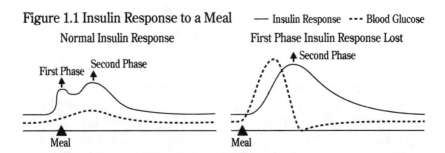

Figure 1.1 Insulin Response to a Meal — Insulin Response --- Blood Glucose

Normal Insulin Response   First Phase Insulin Response Lost

So without her first-phase insulin response, Helen is now beginning to cross over into diabetes territory. As her blood sugars climb, they tend to stay up. This is because it takes more insulin to conquer a high than to maintain a normal blood sugar. Once the blood sugars start to go up, gradually increasing a little at a time, they will stay up. One year Helen's fasting blood sugar might be in the 90s and after meals in the 130s to 140s. A couple

---

*Blood sugar numbers refer to milligrams (mg) of glucose per deciliter (dl) of blood We use the term "points" for simplification. Thus, 20 points would be 20 mg/dl and 40 points would be 40 mg/dl.

of Thanksgiving and Christmas celebrations later, she'll get fasting readings running 100–110 and get up to 150–160 after meals. It's something that just sneaks up on you little by little.

The phenomenon in which Helen's insulin doesn't work as well to conquer high sugars as it does to handle normal ones is called glucose toxicity. Blood sugar levels of 150–180 are considered toxic, because that's where the trouble that causes complications begins. These are the kinds of blood sugars that will lead to the fatigue, skin problems, and tinglings that will eventually cause Helen to go to the doctor.

Helen is now into full-blown diabetes but she doesn't know it. And that third problem we talked about before is setting in. Her insulin resistance is now so great that the cells in her liver that are supposed to notice all that insulin in her bloodstream have totally lost their ability to detect it. In the middle of the night after four or five hours of nothing to eat, her liver's job is to start putting glucose in her bloodstream as her blood sugar drops. The liver is a storage tank of fuel so that we never run out, even when we don't eat. Helen's liver, since it can't detect the presence of insulin in her bloodstream (its signal that there's food there), goes berserk. It pours out lots and lots of glucose. Helen gets excessive liver glucose production and delivery in the night, so she gets up in the morning with high blood sugar. That high morning blood sugar means she'll be high all day long, since her insulin no longer has the ability to bring down high blood sugars. When she finally goes to the doctor and has a blood sugar test, she'll find out why she doesn't feel well anymore.

JUNE AND BARBARA: We just hope she goes to the doctor sooner rather than later, because the longer she waits, the higher her blood sugars will go. We do have one word of comfort, at least for people who are older than Helen—say, in their 70s. Dr. Peter Forsham, professor emeritus in medicine and pediatrics at the University of California at San Francisco (who has had diabetes for 67 years), said in a lecture we heard that damage from high blood sugar doesn't usually begin for the elderly until levels over 200.

Now that we see the formidable problems with Type II-R's, how about June and her lean (but not mean unless their blood sugar gets too low) Type II-D cohorts? What makes them the way they are?

VIRGINIA: We've all seen some adults with diabetes who do not fit the picture we have been painting about insulin resistance. Do they have Type II diabetes? Yes and no. Yes, it is Type II as we currently define it, but they are not insulin-resistant, hyperinsulinemic types. They are lean at the time of diagnosis and generally can't be controlled with the oral hypoglycemic agents (bloodsugar–lowering pills). They are not insulin resistant, because they can control their blood glucose with small doses of insulin, but they do require those small doses. Sometimes we call them Type I 1/2, but for this book, as we've said, we'll call them Type II-D for insulin-deficient.

June and her cohorts really are a forgotten minority in the diabetes world, but they do have an advantage. They seem to do well in avoiding the complications of diabetes.

JUNE AND BARBARA: Shucks, we thought that June was complication-free after 25 years of diabetes because she was so meticulous in her self-care. Maybe she should lighten up a little.

VIRGINIA: No, don't do that! Good care plays a major role in avoiding complications for *all* people with diabetes. It's just that having some insulin on board seems to be a protective feature. Type II-D's also don't have excessive insulin floating around their bloodstreams to cause cardiovascular risk as the Type II-R's do. They also seem to be able to control their blood glucose more easily than a "true" Type I, because, unlike Type I's, they are not totally insulin deficient. Still, they do have the challenges of multiple insulin injections and testing their blood sugars daily and, of course, watching their diet.

JUNE AND BARBARA: How do you know the Type II-D's are still making some insulin of their own?

VIRGINIA: We know because they rarely, if ever, go into diabetic coma, or, as we say in medical circles, ketoacidosis (often abbreviated DKA). DKA is caused by extremely high blood sugars from lack of insulin. The Type II-D's are protected from DKA because they still make some insulin, at least enough so that some glucose can get into their cells and prevent the body from sending out the message that it's starving. That message tells the body to start breaking down fat and converting it to glucose. When this happens, the conversion of fat and protein to glucose leaves a waste product called ketones. These are acid products that are very bad for your body. When your acid-base balance is upset, your normal metabolic processes cannot work. This is a serious medical crisis that calls for immediate hospitalization. Typically, Type I diabetics will report that especially at times of stress from illness they've had bouts of DKA. But it is unusual for an adult lean Type II-D to experience DKA, and if it does happen, it's usually at a time of extreme stress, such as a surgery.

JUNE AND BARBARA: What causes this not-very-common type of diabetes that June has?

VIRGINIA: Researchers haven't even classified it yet, but it is probably like Type I, only it's slower and, because it strikes later in life, it is less devastating to the beta cells of the pancreas. Type II-D is probably inherited in the same fashion as Type I. With Type I there is a genetic set-up for susceptibility, but some additional environmental triggers are required for the disease to develop. It does not strike everyone in the family even though they have the same genetic framework. Obviously, then, there are additional factors at work. Many researchers believe that one or more viral onslaughts for people with the diabetic genetic set-up cause their immune system to be fooled into thinking that their own beta cells are bad guys. The immune system destroys the beta cells over a period of several years. Someday, hopefully we will be able to detect this process early enough to stop the immune system damage and prevent Type I diabetes.

This is a very different scenario from Type II diabetes, which does not appear to be related to a viral/immune system process. Type II is also a genetic disease, but it seems to strike a much higher rate of family members who have the susceptibility. In studies of identical twins, in cases where one twin gets Type I diabetes, 40 to 50 percent of the identical siblings get the disease;

when one twin gets Type II, 90 percent of the identical siblings become diabetic.

JUNE AND BARBARA: In your introduction, Virginia, you told us that Type II diabetes in overweight people is caused by a metabolic error they are born with. Most people know that diabetes is a genetic disease, but they may not know about this other genetic disorder. This one has to do with the way food is metabolized (converted to energy). This disorder explains why being overweight and getting Type II diabetes go together. And they do go together, because between 80 and 90 percent of Type II's are overweight. Can you describe the metabolic error that accounts for the initial weight problem of most Type II's, a problem that is later exacerbated by excess insulin production?

VIRGINIA: To understand this disorder we have to go back to our origins in this country—to the tribes of Native Americans who were here in the first place. I said that between 6 and 10 percent of the U.S. population has diabetes, but that's the overall figure. In Native Americans, Hispanics, and blacks the incidence of diabetes is more than 10 percent. Diabetes favors minorities, and the most favored of all are Native American citizens.

Native Americans are as much as 300 times more likely to get diabetes than Anglos. The professionals who work with the Indian Health Service explain this extraordinary rate of diabetes with the "thrifty gene" theory. This theory starts with the plight of the Indians a few thousand years ago. Imagine yourself living in America as a Zuni or a Sioux. You work from morning until night to get enough food to survive. Your food consists of fruits and berries gathered and perhaps corn grown in poor irrigation conditions. Your meat is lean wild game. Your life is one of strenuous hard work, and starvation is a major cause of death. Some persons evolve a metabolism that is very efficient and can "store" a higher percentage of food than other people. These are the people who will live through the winter, because they use less of their food for energy and store more of what they eat for times of famine. These are the ones who reproduce and pass on their life-saving metabolism.

JUNE AND BARBARA: That doesn't sound like a metabolic error, but more like a metabolic advantage.

VIRGINIA: Then was then and now is now. The advantage changes into a disadvantage when you take these people into the 20th century. Give them cars and all the food they want, especially a diet high in fat (fat foods are stored as fat in the body more quickly than protein or carbohydrate foods), and you have people who gain weight very easily, coupled with a built-in genetic tendency toward Type II diabetes. These people have both insulin resistance and a metabolism designed to survive famine. With a body programmed like this, it's a real challenge to overcome civilization. After all, it has only been a few generations of Native Americans who have enjoyed ample food and modern transportation. And now we have to tell our Native American friends with diabetes to eat less and walk more. It's not surprising that many of them think we've lost our minds.

With this genetic double-whammy, the Indian people in America are being devastated by diabetes. In many tribes, as many as half of the adults have Type II diabetes. Among Native Americans, gestational diabetes (a form that emerges during pregnancy) occurs in as many as 20 percent of pregnancies, compared to 3 percent in the rest of the population. This will only perpetuate the cycle. Amputations and kidney failure are occurring in the Native American population at rates that stagger the imagination. A couple of summers ago I visited the Hualapai tribe near the Grand Canyon in Arizona. This village of 1,500 people has a kidney failure rate 1,000 times greater than the national average.

Recently I was in Sacaton, Arizona, and had the opportunity to meet many of the Pima people, 50 percent of whom have diabetes. Let me tell you about Joy. She is 36 years old and has had diabetes for three years. It's not uncommon to find Pima children 8 and 10 years old with *Type II* diabetes. I talked with Joy about getting better control of her blood glucose levels without having to go on insulin. She's already at the maximum dose of oral hypoglycemics. She was very receptive to trying a Fast Fast (carbohydrate-restricted diet; see Chapter 4) for a few days and then working on her diet, although I must tell you she was already doing most things right.

She told me she does not allow any cookies or chips in her house and wants to make sure her children eat right so that they don't get diabetes. That made me very sad, because it is not chips and cookies that are going to give her children diabetes. Of course, no one needs chips and cookies (except in rare emergencies), but we must not blame the disease on the patient. Joy will help her children eat better and live longer, because they're working on low-fat and high-fiber eating patterns. For example, a group on the reservation is involved in a project called The Native Seeds/SEARCH. SEARCH stands for Southwestern Endangered Aridlands Resource Clearing House. It is one of the country's first regional seed banks, founded to keep ancient desert plants and traditional farming methods from disappearing. The group has been collecting and researching traditional diets and working to reintroduce life-saving foods into Native American diets. I tasted the tepary beans at the group's booth at a local health fair. Cooked without any fat or salt, they tasted better than any other beans I've eaten. (You can write for their catalog at Native Seeds/SEARCH, 2509 N. Campbell Ave., #325, Tucson, AZ 85719. Native Americans get free seeds and the rest of us can buy them inexpensively.)

For the sake of Joy's children and all the Pima children, I hope we will find the answer to prevent and cure this disease. All the Pima people I met are very concerned about their health and the well-being of their families. It's very disturbing to see the level of devastation that diabetes is causing in these lovely people.

JUNE AND BARBARA: These figures are genuinely frightening. We can only hope that the Indian Health Service will tackle this problem with all possible government resources and then some. We heard Dr. Harold E. Lebovitz, author of *Newer Concepts of Type II Diabetes* and professor of medicine and chief of endocrinology and diabetes at Down State Medical Center in New York, tell a conference that 25 to 45 percent of American Indians now have diabetes. He also emphasized the prevalence of diabetes among the Hispanic population—between 13 and 14 percent. Even more appalling, 30 to 40 percent of Hispanic women over age 55 have diabetes. Why do Hispanic people also have such a high rate of diabetes?

VIRGINIA: This is an interesting question, because if you go back to the Spanish ancestors of today's Hispanics, you do not find an increased rate of diabetes. The Spanish explorers who came to America brought a rich cultural heritage and horses, and some say they brought venereal disease, but it seems they did not bring diabetes to America. The Hispanic people of Mexico and the Southwest often forget that their Spanish ancestors who populated the area in the 1600s did not bring any women with them. Their high rate of diabetes is a genetic heirloom from the local Indian people with whom the Spanish mingled and married. People of Hispanic descent in America are 10 to 15 times more likely to develop diabetes than the Anglo population. Most of them will get Type II diabetes, although there are Hispanic people who have Type I.

JUNE AND BARBARA: That brings us to America's black population. Ten percent of black Americans suffer from diabetes and it's the third leading cause of death in their racial group. An article in the February 1991 *Diabetes Forecast* explained that the high occurrence of obesity among blacks contributes greatly to this. And the main reason for their high rate of obesity (60 percent of black women over 45 years of age are obese) is poverty and the diet that poverty imposes on them. Thirty-four percent of black men and women are below the poverty line, while only about 11 percent of white men and women are. Poverty and obesity, as the article puts it, often go together. Blacks also have "thrifty" genes because they're descended from Africans who had to hunt for food just like the early Native Americans did.

And now, Virginia, we finally come to people like you. You have those "thrifty" genes but you're an Anglo. Where do you fit in?

VIRGINIA: True, I'm not a Native American, even though I was raised in Oklahoma, nor am I Hispanic or black, but I got diabetes at a young age, just as some of the populations with high rates of diabetes do. In fact, they're getting it at younger and younger ages. I have a Norwegian grandmother and I have diabetes on both sides of my family. Lots of Northern European peoples developed the same "efficient" metabolism that allowed them to survive feast-and-famine lifestyles. In fact, Type II diabetes is increasing in the general population of the United States at the rate of 6 percent a year.

This brings me to something I heard the other day that goes along with this discussion of how Type II diabetes is Mother Nature's way of maintaining the species. An overweight Type II diabetic named Frank came into our center. Frank had been a prisoner of war in World War II, and when we explained to him how Type II diabetes works and why he has the problems he does, he got this sudden enlightened look on his face. "So that's why I never lost weight in the prison camp!" he exclaimed.

He went on to tell us how he had been in the camp for almost a year and was about the same weight when he came out as when he went in, while his comrades were reduced to skin and bones. He said, "Granted, I did get a little more food than my buddies did because I could speak Italian. I would go over and talk to the Italian prisoners and they would sometimes slip me a little pasta or something. But I certainly didn't get anywhere near the kind of food I needed, and yet I hardly lost any weight at all. I always wondered about that."

This is an excellent illustration of the fact that simply decreasing calories is not the way to lose weight. A low-calorie diet alone is absolutely not going to help the person with Type II diabetes. You see, the other aspect of being a prisoner of war was that Frank got almost no exercise, being confined to a small space.

What we're doing now with Frank is first working on having him cut down the amount of fat he's eating. But I've told him what I have to tell all Type II diabetics: his chances of getting down to an ideal body weight are two—a slim chance and no chance at all. So you see, it's especially important that we set other goals for ourselves: the goals of being healthy and fit. Fit means normal levels of blood sugar, normal blood lipids (the blood fats that can cause heart disease), normal blood pressure, and normal amounts of exercise in our lives. We should be able to walk and work and play and feel good. That's what's important.

JUNE AND BARBARA: Since you've mentioned blood pressure, that gives us a chance to ask about another unpleasant statistic having to do with Type II diabetes. To us it's astounding that between 45 and 50 percent of Type II's also have high blood pressure, and this is regardless of their ethnic background. How do you account for this and what does it mean?

VIRGINIA: It means that diabetes is more and more being recognized, not as a single disease, but as part of a group of diseases and possibly even the cause of all the diseases in the group. This larger problem is sometimes mysteriously called Syndrome X or, more descriptively, insulin resistance syndrome. I call it "hyperbetes," because its main features are hypertension and diabetes. Hypertension is the scientific word for high blood pressure.

I know this is a book about Type II diabetes, but we must look at the bigger picture. Over half of the people with Type II either have or will get high blood pressure. The other diseases of Syndrome X are hyperlipidemia and atherosclerotic heart disease. Hyperlipidemia means high levels of fats in the blood, and in this case more is not better. High levels of blood lipids and high blood pressure over time lead to atherosclerotic heart disease (ASHD). This means that the blood vessels that serve the heart are getting clogged up; when one or more of them become totally clogged, it causes a heart attack. People with Type II diabetes die from heart disease more than from any other cause. When I am in the hospital to see patients, I end up spending more time on the heart floors than anywhere else, because over 30 percent of the patients there have diabetes. That is not a coincidence. This is why throughout this book we'll be talking about treating diabetes, but it may sound like we're treating heart disease instead.

JUNE AND BARBARA: We see there's a lot more to worry about than we realized and that we need to understand serious health problems other than diabetes. Why don't you take these terms—hypertension, hyperlipidemia, and atherosclerotic heart disease—and define each of them for us before we go on?

VIRGINIA: Hypertension simply means high blood pressure. Normal blood pressure is about 120/80. Blood pressure over 140/90 is considered elevated. Hyperlipidemia means that you have high levels of lipids (fatty substances) in your blood. Blood lipids consist of triglycerides, cholesterol, and phospholipids. These circulate in your blood and are hooked up to proteins.

That's why you may hear your doctor refer to them as lipoproteins. So now you may be asking, what are triglycerides and cholesterol?

Triglycerides: These are the main storage form of lipids and constitute about 95 percent of the fatty tissue of the body.

Cholesterol: This is a natural component of cell membranes and is used to make other substances in the body, such as some hormones. Cholesterol can be absorbed from food or it can be manufactured by the liver. The kinds of cholesterol you hear about are HDL (high-density lipoprotein) and LDL (low-density lipoprotein). HDLs are known as "good lipids" because they are associated with decreased risk of heart disease. LDLs are known as "bad lipids" because a high level of LDLs has a strong and direct association with coronary artery disease. So you see, it is not enough to have a good total cholesterol anymore (under 200). You have to have high HDLs (above 50) and low LDLs (below 130).

Atherosclerotic heart disease: I've pretty much already described this one as fat-clogged blood vessels that can cause a heart attack. The problems that contribute to ASHD are diabetes, high blood lipids, high blood pressure, and smoking. Smoking more than doubles your risk of ASHD and it is something you can choose to do or not. So don't do it!

JUNE AND BARBARA: Besides not smoking, what can you do about "hyperbetes"?

VIRGINIA: Hypertension and high blood lipids will improve if you follow our recommendation of a low-fat, low-salt diet and exercise. But remember that these problems are genetic and if they don't get better with lifestyle changes, there are excellent medications that will help. Check with your doctor regarding your goal range for lipids and have them checked at least twice a year. Have your blood pressure checked at least every three months and have a goal of a systolic number (that's the top number) of less than 130 and a diastolic number (that's the bottom one) as close to 80 as possible. This is referred to as 130 over 80.

There are newer and better drugs for treating high blood pressure these days. They are classified as calcium channel blockers and ACE (angiotensin converting enzyme) inhibitors. They have been found to be especially beneficial for people with diabetes in that they may have a protective effect on the kidneys. Check with your doctor about whether these drugs would be suited for you. Also, blood pressure medication is like diabetes medication in the sense that you may need it for a while and then with weight loss and exercise, you may be able to discontinue it. That's why it's important to see your doctor and get your blood pressure checked every three months so that he or she can adjust your dose as needed.

As you can see, "hyperbetes" is something we can all live with. One of our patients, Celia, is a good example. She came to us with all the classic symptoms. She had diabetes with a glycohemoglobin of 10+, (see page 35 for a definition), she was about 70 pounds overweight, and she had high blood pressure and elevated lipids. She had the hypertension part of the syndrome before the diabetes. At least, it was diagnosed first. She was put on a diuretic (water pill) for the high blood pressure and it did what diuretics often do—it raised her blood sugar. This is one of the reasons that diuretics are not the best drug group for treating high blood pressure in people with diabetes.

Celia was sent to us for diabetes education, and we realized that the diuretic was probably the culprit. We suggested she consult one of our endocrinologists. Our docs put her on a better regimen of blood-pressure-lowering medication plus oral agents for her diabetes. After a few months of working with our dietitians for diabetes control, she lost 22 pounds and was able to stop taking her blood-pressure medication, her lipid-lowering drugs, and her diabetes pills. So you see, the diabetes lifestyle—low-fat diet, weight loss, exercise—works to treat the "hyperbetes" syndrome. Celia was thrilled, and we'll continue to work with her to stay in good control.

Don't get me wrong. There is nothing wrong with medications for treating blood pressure, lipids, and diabetes. We would all prefer to get along without them, and often early in the disease that is possible. But when it is not possible, it's important to follow the prescribed treatment.

CHAPTER 2

Ways and Means of Control: Doing What You Have to Do

Now we come to the major un-fun part of diabetes—the tedious part, the boring part, the relentless, day-after-day part. This is the testing of your blood sugar to see where you are and, in some cases, the taking of pills or insulin to get you where you want to be and keep you there.

Faced with this most unsatisfying aspect of diabetes, we need a little shot of philosophy. How about this one from Thomas Merton's *The Springs of Contemplation; A Retreat at the Abbey of Gethsemani:*

"If I insist that my work ... mustn't be tedious or monotonous, I'm in trouble. ... Time after time it fails to become so. So I get more agitated about it, I fight with people about it. I make more demands about it. It's ridiculous to demand that work always be pleasurable, because work is not necessarily pleasing. ... If we're detached and simply pick up the job we have to do and go ahead and do it, it's usually fairly satisfying. Even jobs that are repugnant and dull or tedious tend to be quite satisfying, once we get right down to doing them. This happens when we just do what we have to do."

That's the way it is with doing what we sometimes refer to as "diabetic shenanigans." June tests her blood sugar six or seven times a day and takes five separate injections—sometimes more if she's sick or changing time zones or her blood sugars have gone haywire for some other reason. If she got agitated and fought with people about having to do this, she'd be a one-woman war zone. No, she just does what she has to do.

It's not likely that you'll have this much tedium and travail in your diabetic life, especially if you're a Type II-R, but you still need to do what you have to do. And if you just do it without agitation, you'll find it's not so bad, maybe even quite satisfying, especially when you discover that you did what you had to do—and it worked!

There's another advantage to doing your diabetic shenanigans. It helps you keep your mind alert and your wits about you. Chief Justice Oliver Wendell Holmes, who lived to be 94, kept his mind sharp right up to the end by doing crossword puzzles every day. Being diabetic means never having to look around for an activity to keep you on your mental toes. You've got one built in that will last your whole life.

So now Virginia will do what she has to do—show you what you have to do and how to do it so you can go forth and just do it!

—June and Barbara

What You'll Find in This Chapter

Goals for Blood Sugar Levels
Choosing a Doctor
Glycohemoglobin Test
Urine and Blood Sugar Testing
Keeping Records
Medication: Pills and Insulin
Buying Supplies

JUNE AND BARBARA: What do health professionals mean when they say a person with diabetes is "in control" or "out of control"?

VIRGINIA: This refers to how closely their blood sugars align with what their blood sugar goals are. Goals are established individually for each person. For instance, for a person who is nearing 80 years of age we don't need goals that aim for tight control (mostly normal blood sugars). Tight control is ideally designed to prevent complications down the road. When you're 80 the complications that you fear 30 years from the time of diagnosis are pretty insignificant. You can settle for blood sugars in a range where you feel good. No matter what your age, you deserve to feel good!

Again, in an elderly person severe hypoglycemia (low blood sugar) should be avoided because it can be dangerous. It could lead to a serious fall, for example. Depending on the individual, we might extend the goal range to somewhat higher than the tighter control levels generally recommended for younger people. We keep in mind, though, that if blood sugars go too high, the elderly person will not feel good and will be at increased risk of dehydration and infections.

The goals we would suggest for young people and children (not many Type II's are in this age group) would be different. We might suggest the normal range of fasting blood sugars of 70–120 and one hour after meals of 100–140. We'd want to consider that this person has 40, 50, or 60 years to live with this disease and we'd like to prevent complications.

For most Type II adults—the neither very young nor very old—we're happy with a before-breakfast blood sugar in the neighborhood of 80–140 and after-meal blood sugars less than 180–200. Those are what we call near-normal ranges; in other words, close enough to normal to prevent complications, yet not so close to normal that we're constantly battling hypoglycemia if the person is on medication.

Some Type II's on insulin have severe hypoglycemic reactions with little or no warning. This sometimes happens to those who've had diabetes a long time. They lose their ability to sense the reactions. This is called hypoglycemic unawareness. Most diabetics can recognize an insulin reaction because of the typical symptoms of shaking, sweating, dizziness, poor coordination, and even less dramatic signs such as hunger, blurred vision, and irritability.

People who've developed hypoglycemic unawareness don't have these warning symptoms. They can get such a low blood sugar level that they suddenly pass out. This is why we tell them that it is their responsibility to test their blood sugar before they get behind the steering wheel of a car. Every time! And it should always be above 120 before they start out.

JUNE AND BARBARA: When people are first diagnosed—and even sometimes later on down the line—they often ask, "How do I go about finding a physician who's really good at managing diabetes?"

VIRGINIA: My advice would be to ask other people with diabetes and get their recommendations. If you don't know any other diabetics (not likely these days!) you could call your local diabetes association and ask for the names of some doctors specializing in diabetes. If you don't have a local diabetes association, you could call a local hospital and ask which physicians on their staff specialize in diabetes. One thing to watch for when you're doctor-shopping is to find one who has a team of diabetes educators at his disposal. A doctor who does not use diabetes educator nurses and dietitians is not serious about managing diabetes.

JUNE AND BARBARA: Most people already have a family doctor, and so their question is likely to be, "Is it OK to stay with my family doctor to take care of my diabetes or do I need to go to an expert such as an endocrinologist or diabetologist?" Before you answer that, for the uninitiated, you'd better clarify exactly what these two specialists are and what they do.

VIRGINIA: An endocrinologist is an internal medicine physician who has had additional training in endocrine diseases (those involving the secretion of various hormones). Usually he has had an additional two-year fellowship and will probably be board certified in endocrinology. (Tip: Read the diplomas and certificates on the office wall.) Over half of the patients of most endocrinologists have diabetes. It's by far the most common endocrine problem. Some endocrinologists refer to themselves as diabetologists because they specialize in the care of diabetes. A diabetologist can also be an internal medicine physician who did not take a fellowship in endocrinology but who specializes in diabetes in his practice.

JUNE AND BARBARA: Now that we know what endocrinologists and diabetologists are, let's go back to the basic question: "Do I need one?"

VIRGINIA: That's a question each individual has to decide for himself or herself. But there's help available in making your decision: the standards-of-care criteria written by the American Diabetes Association. These standards were developed by a consensus of top medical minds in diabetes and were designed to assure the best quality of care and also be cost effective. They are available from your local ADA affiliate (call them and ask for reprint #CAIS335, which costs 45 cents). After reading them, you may ask yourself, "Am I getting this kind of monitoring of my progress and is my family physician capable of providing this level of monitoring?" If your answer is yes and you feel you have a good relationship with your doctor and are getting the continuity of care that is so important for a person with a chronic disease, then very likely you'll do fine with the doctor you have. It is also important, however, for you to have access to diabetes educators either through your doctor's office or elsewhere in the community.

On the other hand, an endocrinologist offers a different level of expertise in analyzing and treating the endocrine problems that you may be experiencing. You may need such help especially when you're just starting out your life as a diabetic. An initial consultation with an endocrinologist can get you off on the right track for the best level of care and diabetes control.

Many people will decide to stay with the endocrinologist either because they have difficulty in achieving control or because their care is complicated by another problem such as hypertension or a thyroid disorder, and they need the additional level of expertise of the endocrinologist in these areas.

Another time that an endocrinologist may be especially valuable is when you have had diabetes for many years and are starting to experience complications or are worried that you might develop them. In either case, you might need the services of an endocrinologist for complication screening and treatment.

JUNE AND BARBARA: Is it an either/or situation? Once you decide to work with an endocrinologist, must you say farewell to your family doctor and the long-time relationship you've built up with him or her?

VIRGINIA: Not at all. As I said before, you may feel you need an endocrinologist at the beginning and then, after you feel confident that your diabetes is in control and you can handle it, you can go back to your family doctor.

Then, too, you can be under the care of a primary-care physician and use an endocrinologist as a consultant who only works with you on your diabetes problems. Your family doctor is the one who takes care of your everyday sniffles and sore throats and flus and your other general medical problems. This is the best solution for many people.

JUNE AND BARBARA: Is the best solution always possible? Doesn't your health insurance provider or your HMO tell you what you have to do when it comes to seeking help for your diabetes?

VIRGINIA: That's true. Many times the third-party payment systems require that you go to your primary-care physician for basic care, and they only let you see an endocrinologist if your primary-care physician thinks it's necessary and gives you a referral to one.

JUNE AND BARBARA: What happens when you think you need to consult an endocrinologist and your primary-care physician thinks you don't?

VIRGINIA: Although that sounds like an impossible tug-of-war for you, there is someone available to put some weight on your end of the rope. Health maintenance organizations have care managers or benefit supervisors to help resolve such situations. They may negotiate with your primary-care physician to give you at least an initial referral or they may even assign you to a different primary-care physician. This latter might be the best idea, since if the disagreement has gone this far, it may have undermined the doctor-patient relationship to the point that you can no longer work effectively together.

Let me emphasize something here: It doesn't pay to be shy when it comes to your personal health care needs. Nobody is giving nice-guy points when it comes to taking care of your own health needs. You must realize too that no one—health professional or not—will take the level of responsibility for your health care that you yourself will. It is especially important for you to develop this attitude of self-responsibility in this day and age when all of the health care systems are looking for the most cost-effective ways to deliver health care. You have to be strong, capable, and well-informed if you want the care you need and deserve.

JUNE AND BARBARA: That reminds us of our friend Jean, a college professor. She was in the hospital several days for extensive tests. Whenever she felt the care she received was inept or ineffective, she let the hospital staff know about it in no uncertain terms and demanded that the situation be rectified *immediately*. She almost always got what she wanted. As she was leaving the hospital, and had mellowed out somewhat because of the favorable results of her stay, she remarked to a nurse, "I guess I'm known around here as the scourge of the fifth floor."

"No," replied the nurse, smiling sweetly, "the scourge of the whole west wing."

Now, being obnoxious in general just because you're unhappy at being sick or incapacitated doesn't help matters in health care any more than it does in any other area of life. But we agree with Virginia (and know from our own experience) that a little scourging at the right time can work wonders when you are being denied the care—or the endocrinologist—that you know you need.

Before we leave the realm of the endocrinologist, is there any other time in life when a person with diabetes might require the services of one?

VIRGINIA: Absolutely! During pregnancy. Any woman with diabetes who is even thinking about having a baby should be under the care of an endocrinologist. In the first place, you want to be in good diabetes control *before* getting pregnant, since most of the damage the baby might receive from a mother with out-of-control diabetes takes place in the first trimester. Then, after you become pregnant, you'll probably also want to work with a perinatologist, a physician who specializes in high-risk obstetrics. If you can find a diabetes pregnancy team, this is the most effective way to manage the problems of diabetes and pregnancy. The "dream team" would consist of (1) an endocrinologist, (2) a perinatologist, (3) an obstetrician, (4) a diabetes nurse educator, (5) a diabetes dietitian educator, (6) a genetic counselor, and (7) a social worker. Call your local diabetes association to find such a diabetes and pregnancy program. It's certainly more complicated for a woman with diabetes to have a baby, but with the proper care and attention on her part and on the part of the health professionals she works with, she can have a healthy, happy baby just like any other woman.

JUNE AND BARBARA: Lots of doctors don't seem all that interested in their patients' daily blood sugar tests. They act as if the only really important thing is the glycohemoglobin (hemoglobin A1c) test . Maybe you should explain what this laboratory test is and why doctors consider it so important.

VIRGINIA: I've known physicians who consider the glycohemoglobin to be the most important—if not the only important—test for their patients. To put it simply, this test analyzes how much glucose has bonded with your red blood cells and, thereby, indicates what your average blood sugars have been for the past 8 to 10 weeks (the time varies from individual to individual). It's a test that must be attended to since it most closely aligns with risks for the complications of diabetes. This makes it an extremely important indicator; a kind of shining beacon to the person with diabetes to illuminate what the future may hold. Certainly we all want to pay attention to the results of this test, to understand what it means, and, above all, to strive to stay within 10–15 percent of the top of the normal range.

It's important for you to understand that in your glycohemoglobin test you don't necessarily have to get within the normal range for your particular lab value. That normal range is where people who don't have diabetes generally fall. If you're within 10 to 15 percent of normal, that is probably an acceptable level. For example, if the normal range in the test you're taking is 4–6 and your glycohemoglobin is 7, that's great, a good range. When you get up close to 8, that's still OK, but not exquisite. Over 9, we're getting into the terrible range.

One problem with glycohemoglobin tests is that labs around the country vary in the numbers and in the process they use to do the tests. Consequently, numbers that are in the normal range in one lab's test, may be abnormally high—or low—in another's.

JUNE AND BARBARA: That's certainly true. June recently took two glycohemoglobin tests. In one the "normal" range was 5.9 to 7.5 and in the other it was 3.6 to 6.0.

VIRGINIA: That is why you must ask your doctor what is the normal range for the particular test you're taking and what your personal range should be.

If it's the glycohemoglobin test that is so important, why bother doing daily blood sugars? Because you can't fix a poor glycohemoglobin result unless you know what your daily blood sugars are—day in and day out—and work to improve those.

To sum it up: the glycohemoglobin test is your long-term beacon. Your blood sugar tests tell you how you're doing in controlling your diabetes on a day-to-day basis. The daily tests give you the clues as to where your control problems are and what you need to do to improve. These two tests go hand in hand like love and marriage. Both are absolutely necessary if you want really good control.

JUNE AND BARBARA: Some people with diabetes are first told to test the amount of sugar in their urine in order to help with their control (this is the old-fashioned way), while others are put directly onto blood sugar testing. What is the difference between testing urine and blood?

VIRGINIA: It's very simple: Urine testing is worthless and blood testing is not. To go into a little more detail, urine glucose measurements are, as you put it, the old-fashioned way. Many years ago when there was no technology available for blood sugar testing at home, urine sugar measurements were thought to give some reflection of blood glucose variations that could be used to keep people in control. Since you don't "spill" (another old-fashioned term) glucose into your urine until your blood sugar is higher than about 180–200 (and even higher than that if you're older), then urine testing isn't going to be of much value. Added to that problem is the fact that urine glucose testing varies with the amount of liquid in the bladder. You may have had a spike of high sugar and then low sugar and you'll still spill glucose in your urine, even though at the time of testing your blood sugar is very low.

Let me give you an analogy. Testing urine for glucose control of diabetes is like driving a car using only the rearview mirror. As far as I'm concerned, it has no value. Some people say, "Yes, but it costs less money." Not really. When you consider the value of the information you get, it's extremely expensive. People also say that it's better than nothing. *Au contraire*. I'd like to assert that it's worse than nothing. Too often you're getting a false sense of security. Many Type II diabetics don't spill glucose into their urine until their blood sugars are in the 300 range (usually older people). As long as they're getting negative urine tests, they think they're doing OK, when in fact they're not.

Did I say urine test strips were worthless? Actually, they do have one useful function. They're great for testing "diet" soft drinks. Did you know that from 10 to 25 percent of fountain "diet" soft drinks may be regular soda instead? One of the teens we take care of did this test at a mall in Albuquerque. He used urine testing strips to test "diet Coke" ordered at all the places where it was available in the mall. More than 10 percent were the real thing and not diet. At one food outlet an employee confessed, "We were out of diet Coke so we hooked up real Coke." Our patient explained to the employee that this deceptive practice could seriously hurt a person with diabetes. You can be sure the employee won't do that again.

JUNE AND BARBARA: We've had lots of people report this nondiet diet drink phenomenon to us. Some who have checked it out have found even higher percentages of "mistakes," up to one-third the wrong thing. You can also use urine test strips to check salad dressings and sauces. If they register below one-half percent glucose on Tes-Tape or Diastix, they're probably safe.

Let's move on now to the subject of blood sugar testing, which is far from worthless.

VIRGINIA: I recommend that our patients do visual strip testing of blood samples. If money is an issue, then we have them cut their test strips in half, so that they use only one strip a day and maybe only three for a whole week. The schedule would be to test your fasting (before-breakfast) blood sugar plus your after-break-fast blood sugar on Monday; on Wednesday test your fasting and your after-lunch sugars; on Friday test before breakfast and after supper. You've used only three strips that entire week, yet you're getting much valuable information. You're getting an idea of how your blood sugars are flowing throughout the week.

JUNE AND BARBARA: Now we've slid gracefully into the next important question. Assuming cost is a prime consideration, at what time of day should people take their blood sugar tests and exactly how often? Different doctors suggest different schedules. Tell us what plan you recommend and why.

VIRGINIA: That depends on what information you need to know. Let me go through the different testing times and what they're telling you. First of all, most of you need to test your fasting blood sugar to find out how you're starting the day. This tells us how you're managing your blood sugar without the impact of food. Since most Type II-R's have high fasting levels (remember that excess liver metabolism phenomenon), even though they may be better off the rest of the day, it's important to know that as well.

Now let's talk about testing after meals. If you really want to know how food is affecting your blood sugars, test an hour to an hour and a half after the meal. This is a true look at how the car-bohydrate is affecting your blood sugar. For people using diet alone to manage their blood sugar, this is important information. Don't expect your post-meal blood sugar to be the same as your fasting. Notice that when I gave you your goals for control there were two different sets, one for fasting and one for after meals. In our center, we like looking at the one-hour number instead of the one-and-a-half-hour number, because it more closely reflects how you're dealing with the food in that meal.

If you're on medication, that's a different story. Many times your doctor has instructed you to test before meals. This is the number you need to know to determine how well the medication is working. For instance, your fasting blood sugar tells you how well the oral hypoglycemic agent you took at supper is working or how well the long-acting insulin that you took last night is working. Many times if you get your fasting blood sugar in the normal range, then the rest of the day works out a lot better. Your before-lunch blood sugar is reflective of both the short-acting insulin that covered breakfast, as well as the long-acting insulin you take to cover the whole day. Sometimes you also have to look at your before-supper blood sugar to get an idea of how you might adjust your morning insulin. It also tells you how well the pill or long-acting insulin you took in the morning is working.

To sum it up for people on medication, probably a before-breakfast and a before-supper test plus an occasional after-meal test would be an adequate schedule. One of the after-meal tests could be done at bedtime. That gives you an idea of how supper is affecting your blood sugar and how well your blood sugar is in control before you go to sleep. If you take long-acting insulin and are very low before bedtime, you need to plan for a snack.

If you're the kind of person who does a lot of strenuous exercise (I hope you are), you should be testing right before your workout. If your blood sugar is below 150, have a snack before you begin your exercise. (The 150 may be a somewhat high or low number for you; it can vary with individuals and the intensity of the exercise.) For those of you on medication, this test is a useful tool to keep you at your best blood sugar level for exercise. Exercise lowers blood sugar. Many people also test after their workout.

You should definitely test if you're feeling the symptoms of low blood sugar (sweating, shaky, nervous, weak, confused). You need to see at what level your blood sugar causes you to have these symptoms of hypoglycemia. Some people get symptoms at

120, while others might not feel low even at 40. Any time you feel hypoglycemic, test to see how low you are and if you really need to eat something.

JUNE AND BARBARA: So far we've only talked about visual test strips—those that you compare to a color chart. Easier to use and much more precise is the system where the strip is put in a meter that analyzes it and gives the result as a digital readout. There must be 10 or 12 models of blood-sugar–testing meters available now from different manufacturers, and new ones seem to be coming on the market every other day. They're all different prices and have many different features. Let's say you're a beginning diabetic, and your health insurance will reimburse you for a meter and the monthly supply of strips to use with it, or that you can afford to pay the expenses yourself. How do you go about acquiring a meter you'll be happy with and trust?

VIRGINIA: Let me give you a few criteria you can use:
1. Buy a meter made by a company you can trust. It doesn't necessarily have to be one of the major manufacturers that's been in business a long time. It could be a young company that's doing a good job of providing a meter system and support. But I'm always a little leery of a brand-new company with a brand-new meter. I can't tell you how many meters have come on the market for a short time, and then disappeared. Some models are shown at conventions for diabetes educators and then never even make it to market. Many of my patients have been stuck with a meter from a company that doesn't support it. By support I mean the company has a tollfree phone number answered by knowledgeable, pleasant, patient customer representatives who are empowered to replace your machine quickly if you're having any problems. Also, they should provide easy-to-understand literature and instructions with the machine.
2. Buy a meter system that requires little or no operator technique. As far as I'm concerned, the easiest systems are those that do not require you to wipe the drop of blood off the test pad at a certain moment after you put it on. There are good

systems out there—in fact, they're into second or third generation—that use wipeless strips. These advanced, leading-edge meters sometimes cost more than the old-fashioned meters. But don't be foolish and try to save 25 bucks up front on your purchase if it means you're going to be stuck with a system that requires careful technique and, therefore, has a lot of error built into it. The strips all cost about the same.

3. Go for a system that supports you in your lifestyle. If you're on the move a lot, go for a system that's small and easy to carry around, easy to use, with easily understood results, and that's accurate. If having a meter in your pocket or purse means you're more likely to do testing, then by all means, get an easily portable machine.

By and large, pharmacists are not experts on meter systems, although some have taken the time and effort to learn about meters. For the most part, pharmacists are experts on drugs and medications; they're not experts on the stuff in front of the counter. So I suggest you talk to a diabetes educator. The educator has training and experience with meters, has spent time out there with people who are actually using meters, and probably knows more about these systems than any other health professional, including your doctor.

JUNE AND BARBARA: Getting all those drops of blood to put on strips is no fun, as you well know. Many people—especially older people—have difficulty. Back when Barbara was teaching the use of meters and found someone who bled easily, she would go into raptures over them. ("You just bleed *wonderfully!* How lucky you are. If only everyone could get blood for their tests as easily as you do, this world would be a better place.") After you get the drop, putting it on the strip correctly can be an even greater ordeal. And when you botch the job, not only have you wasted an expensive strip, but you have to start all over again with a new drop. Do you have any magic solutions for avoiding all of the above bloody mishaps?

VIRGINIA: I don't know if they're magic, but there certainly are solutions. If you're one of those people who don't bleed easily, you should wash your hands in warm water before taking the test. Next, hold your hand down at your side below your hips. If you're sitting in a chair, let your hand hang straight down for a few minutes. This will allow it to fill up with blood.

Some people who have a particularly hard time getting blood find they have to really milk the finger. In this case, it helps if you practice doing this motion the right way. Starting way down at the base of the finger near your hand, milk all the way down the length of the finger to the tip on the palm side of the finger until you get a big drop. Then let go of the finger. Let your finger pink up again, then repeat the milking motion. Some people make the mistake of constantly squeezing the finger, never letting go to allow the blood to come back into the finger.

You should always stick your finger on the sides instead of on the fingerprint surface. The "poochy" sides of your finger actually bleed better. Another thing I suggest is to always stick the underneath side of your finger as opposed to the top side. That way the blood goes onto the strip easily and correctly. If you stick the top side of your finger, the blood tends to drip into your fingernails. This not only makes it hard to get the right amount of blood on the strip, but it's unsightly to walk around with blood under your nails.

The typical textbook on diabetes tells you not to stick in the same place all the time because you will get a callus. Most experienced diabetics know that a callus can be rather welcome because finger pricks in a callus don't hurt. When you get a callus so thick that you can no longer get blood, then you need to move on to other areas.

JUNE AND BARBARA: The well-known diabetic diabetologist Peter Forsham also suggested using this callus technique if you're someone like a musician who's afraid of damaging your fingers with numerous finger-sticks. He advised a concert pianist to take the finger he used least in his playing and always take the test from the same place on that finger, causing a callus to develop there.

June figures that she takes over 2,000 blood sugars a year, but the punctures haven't ruined her fingers in any way. Is this an unusual experience? Do some diabetics have problems with soreness and damaged fingers?

VIRGINIA: Unfortunately some people's fingers get so sore that they can hardly bear the thought of taking another blood sugar. That's why I personally like to stick only the three fingers that have developed calluses thick enough to prevent pain.

But it's also very important to find the right lancing device for you. Some stick way too deep for a particular individual. On the other hand, some don't stick deep enough to get the amount of blood you need for the test. Visit your diabetes educator, who usually has a whole drawer full of them. You can try out several to find the right one.

JUNE AND BARBARA: We've found that the lancet also makes a difference. June has found that even though she uses the same lancing device, some brands of lancets may stick deeper or shallower and some brands are more painful than others.

VIRGINIA: That's certainly true. The new lancets with the triple bevel are much less painful than the others. Although there will undoubtedly soon be other brands of triple-bevel lancets on the market, the one I have found that is remarkably different is the Surelite lancet. It is so much less painful that I never use anything else on myself.

JUNE AND BARBARA: To show how it's truly "different pokes for different folks," June has tried the Surelite and can't get enough blood with it for her test.

VIRGINIA: That's why it's wonderful that there are so many different products on the market. There can be something that works for everyone. When you do find the one that's right for you, stay with it. If you're going to have to stick yourself over and over—and you are!—it's worth any extra pennies you may have to spend to get the lancet that is the least painful.

JUNE AND BARBARA: What if you think the meter you're using just gave you a wrong result—a totally unexpected and inexplicable number? This phenomenon usually only happens with an excessively high result. (We all are usually quite willing to accept low readings as valid.) In the case of the "wrong" reading, the normal reaction is to start cursing the meter. Some people may even want to hurl the thing across the room. Some people may actually do it! What do you suggest doing in such cases?

VIRGINIA: This has certainly happened to all of us. Rather than cursing the meter and throwing it across the room, the first thing you would want to consider is whether this truly could be a meter error. As far as I'm aware, there hasn't been a meter made that won't give you an erroneous number at some point in its life.

To check this out, you should retest, but first you should do some troubleshooting. Check the meter to see if it's clean. Do a control test. A control test means using a drop of control solution that comes with your meter to see if the machine comes up with a number that falls within the acceptable range for the solution. The control test is good for checking both the meter and the strips. The problem is that it costs you a strip to do it.

If your meter has a "check strip," at this point it's a good idea to use one of those. Consider whether the temperature of the meter may be too hot or too cold, because that will affect how it is working. If, for example, the meter has been left in the car and is very warm or very cold to the touch, let it come back to room temperature before you retest. Then retest your blood, being careful that your technique is exactly right and that you're putting the right amount of blood on the strip and doing the timing correctly. This is why I prefer wipeless systems and systems that require very little technique. It's much easier *not* to make mistakes.

At this point, if the reading you get is drastically different from the first one, you have to ask yourself which reading was accurate. One way to do this is to test with a visual testing strip (Chemstrip, Glucose V). This visual test will give you a kind of ballpark reading and you can decide from that which of the drastically different readings is most likely to be the correct one and which was erroneous because of faulty technique.

If, however—as usually happens—both of your meter readings agree fairly closely, then you have to admit to yourself that your blood sugar is indeed in that range, surprising though it may be.

JUNE AND BARBARA: Let's talk about strips and meters and how the costs of both have changed. Back in the olden days when June first started testing her blood sugar, meters were expensive. Her first one, an Ames Eyetone Reflectance Meter, cost $350 *used.* Had she bought a new one, it would have been $650! On the other hand, at that time, strips were relatively inexpensive—45 to 50 cents apiece.

Then the meter manufacturers got onto the razor blade theory. That's the marketing idea Gillette discovered long ago. The razor is sold for very little because the manufacturer knows it then has a long-time customer for its blades, and the blade prices can be on the high side. As a result, meter prices have dropped to as low as $50; sometimes, if you trade in a meter from a rival company, meters are actually free. This is because the makers want you using *their* strips and not the competitors'.

You don't have to be the proverbial rocket scientist to figure out what has happened to strip prices under this scenario. Some of them are now in the 80-cent range and heading north. Back when we were involved with the SugarFree Center, it always gave us a kind of grotesque amusement to see how every year one meter company would raise its strip prices and then—you could almost hear the collective sigh of relief—the other companies would follow suit. Since she tests so frequently, June now spends around $5 a day for strips; in other words, $1,825 a year ($1830 in leap year!). Luckily she has health insurance that reimburses for 80 percent of this cost.

About 10 years ago one company in this country started importing a meter called the Glucochek from England. This meter used a well-known brand of strips made by another company. The meter importing company came out with a device to cut strips in half and an adapter for the meter so it could work with half-strips. This company is no longer in business. They just couldn't survive with the one-time purchase of the meter, adapter, and splitter. And we suspect they may have been legally hassled by the company that made the strips they were encouraging people to cut in half.

At any rate, right now there is no meter that can use half-strips because no manufacturer in its right mind that makes both strips and meters would make a meter that, in effect, cut its profits in half. We've heard of people trying to rig their meters to use strips cut in half or even thirds, but we've never heard of anyone for whom that worked. Virginia, what's your experience with meters and half-strips?

VIRGINIA: The one meter you mentioned that advertised itself as being able to use a half-strip was never very accurate, and I think that actually was the main reason it went out of business. But at this time there is no meter that will work with a half-strip. If you think you're reading a meter with a half-strip, you're just fooling yourself. What does work quite well with a half-strip, though, is visual testing. For people who cannot afford a meter or who cannot afford the meter plus the strips, using a visual Chemstrip cut in half is a good idea. Not only will it save money, but it's actually easier to read a half-strip against the color blocks on the bottle than it is to read a whole strip. On top of that it takes less blood. The way you do it is to cut the strip in half lengthwise. Just cut one at a time; don't do the whole bottle at once. And don't leave the lid off the bottle while you're cutting your strip—you don't want the rest of the strips in the bottle to deteriorate. This is a way to save a lot of money if you have to pay for the strips out of your own pocket. It's particularly good for people who are Type II and not on insulin so their insurance or Medicare will not pay for their strips. Using this method almost everyone can afford to test their blood sugar.

JUNE AND BARBARA: People have often asked us why strips cost so much. Some of them, particularly men with an engineering background, have allowed as how they could go out in the garage and make "a strip like that for about one-quarter cent." Of course, none of them has been able to do this. But they have a point. Why do strips have to be so expensive? Is it just unmitigated greed on the part of the manufacturers?

VIRGINIA: No, I don't think it's even *mitigated* greed. I really don't feel that the companies are ripping off people with diabetes. The technology of blood glucose monitoring has grown tremendously in just 10 years. We've gone from a visual read-only strip to extremely accurate, easy-to-use systems. The costs to develop that new technology and to get FDA approval are exorbitant. Then there are the expenses of packaging, the sales force to spread the word of the new technology and instruct people in its use, advertising, insurance (in this litigious society someone is always trying to sue, especially in the health field), and the ongoing cost of doing the research for the next meter down the line. Companies are starting to work on a noninvasive test (that means you don't have to stick your finger). On top of everything else, the meter and strip companies are generous in their support of diabetes education programs and seminars for professionals and diabetics alike. Actually, I often wonder how they do as well as they do at keeping costs down.

JUNE AND BARBARA: Now that we've worked over the meter and strip companies and the high costs, we have to mention that patients sometimes have unrealistic expectations. One of our favorite stories is of the composer Richard Strauss, who was talking to the casting director for his opera *Salome*. "The woman I want to play the lead role," Strauss said, "should have the lithe body of a nymph and the rich, full voice of a Wagnerian soprano."

"Herr Strauss," said the casting director, shaking his head, "You cannot haff it both vays."

A lot of people, understandably, want to "haff it both vays." They want to purchase their diabetes needs at the rock-bottom prices of a mail-order business using minimum-wage employees operating out of a warehouse in a low-rent area in a far-off state, and they want to purchase them in a place with a pleasant atmosphere, conveniently located not too far from where they live, with a knowledgeable health professional on the job to explain how to use the equipment and answer any questions they may have. And they want to be able to come back for additional help whenever they need it.

Back in the days when we ran the SugarFree Center, quite a few people were having it both ways. We remember our diabetes teaching nurse, Elsie, once spent more than an hour carefully explaining to a woman how all the available meters worked and the advantages of each, so the patient could make an informed decision on what meter to buy. When she finished, the woman said, "The nurse in my doctor's office was right!"

"Right about what?" asked Elsie.

"She said that if I went to the SugarFree Center, you'd show me all the meters and help me choose which one I wanted and then I could run over to Fedco and get it cheap."

Actually sometimes people really want to "haff it three ways." Along with rock-bottom prices and professional assistance in a nice center, they also want an efficient, well-staffed, computerized third-party billing department to file their insurance claims (and wait for the money!) for them.

Given that nobody can have it both (or three) ways, what is your advice in sorting out which of these aspects of care are the most important for most people and how they can do the best they can for themselves while still playing fair with others?

VIRGINIA: I agree that it's a difficult situation. In the end the decision has to be made by the individual based on his or her needs—and his or her conscience. Of course everyone wants to get the best possible price. I have found, though, that if you're learning to monitor your blood sugar for the first time, you should purchase the supplies from someone who can provide individualized education on blood sugar testing in general and on the meter you're purchasing in particular. Some medical supply stores can do this, although sometimes you're getting your instruction from a clerk with no specialized training in patient education or monitors.

Overall, a diabetes educator will probably be your best resource for training, and many times the educator will provide you with a meter or direct you to the best place to get one. Then you can bring the meter in for your training during a visit with the diabetes educator.

It's true that the meter may be cheapest at a mail-order or discount pharmacy. If, however, because of lack of instruction, you do the test wrong and waste strips and get false readings that lead you to taking the wrong amount of medication, the savings wouldn't be worth it!

We've decided at the Diabetes Center that our main business is not selling meters, so we don't try to make a substantial profit on them. But because we include the cost of training from a certified diabetes educator in the price, you can usually get them cheaper at discount stores. We always suggest the discount or mail-order sources to our experienced patients who are upgrading to a newer model or who are buying a spare meter. You shouldn't have to pay for training if you don't need it. Still, it's a good idea to talk to your educator before you order some sensational deal from a catalog. We may be able to tell you why the meter is so cheap (for instance, it may be a meter that they're closing out because a newer and much better model will soon be available) or warn you of potential problems (such as you can only get the strips in Outer Mongolia on the fifth Tuesday of the month).

So my advice is to get your initial training from a diabetes educator and look for cheaper sources for subsequent meters.

JUNE AND BARBARA: One thing we've noticed is that people often don't want to pay for diabetes education. They're willing to buy equipment and supplies because those are things they can hold in their hands and carry out the door. But in reality the most valuable commodity they can buy is a better understanding of diabetes care. There's a Chinese proverb that we particularly like: "Put your money in your head, and nobody can take it away from you."

Part of the problem may be that insurance companies are sometimes reluctant to pay for education. This is a penny-wise and pound-foolish approach, since a well-educated diabetes patient is more likely to stay out of the hospital where they'll run up huge bills for the insurance company to cover.

VIRGINIA: I couldn't agree more! Many studies have shown clearly that patient education pays off in terms of reduced hospitalizations and better health outcomes for the person with diabetes. But insurance companies, Medicare, and Medicaid are very inconsistent in their payment track record when it comes to diabetes education. The American Diabetes Association implemented a system of rigorous national standards for diabetes education programs. They have "recognized" (approved) over 200 programs. Believe me, it's tough to get "recognized." We found that our center was a better one for having gone through the process. (Call your local American Diabetes Association office to find a recognized diabetes education program in your area.)

The ADA made this effort so that health insurance companies would know which programs to reimburse, but so far, in most places, there has not been any change. I feel that with enough pressure from the public, insurance companies will recognize the value of diabetes education. As the public demands more involvement in their own health and as prevention takes precedence over treatment, I think diabetes education will become increasingly important and insurance will start reimbursing.

JUNE AND BARBARA: Is keeping records of your blood sugar tests absolutely essential? Recording the results is a lot of trouble, and what good is it—especially if you keep getting more-or-less the same numbers and they're all too high? We've had people show us their records and have been amazed that day in and day out they'll write down the same 240s, 280s, or 310s and not question the pointlessness of keeping track of the same bad blood sugars without getting the message that *something different has to be done.* Surely blood sugar testing isn't an end in itself.

VIRGINIA: I agree that keeping records of blood sugars without taking any action is pointless. But I really encourage patients to keep track of their blood sugars while they are coming in for consultations with the diabetes educators. These records can help them identify areas of behavior that are causing them problems. For instance, we can correlate the high blood sugars with changes in diet, medication, or exercise. Also, by identifying patterns in the blood sugar readings we can help them change their medication to correct the problems.

But most importantly, while we're reviewing the records of their food intake, their blood sugars, and their exercise, we can help them learn our decision-making process. This is most important. Fine-tuning diabetes control is not rocket science. It's just being very sensitive to a person's lifestyle. We're never judgmental about blood sugars and we teach the patients not to be judgmental either. Blood sugars don't have anything to do with a person's character. They simply represent the effects of medication, exercise, food, and lifestyle on that particular individual. With time and practice you can learn how to make the adjustments in these factors just as well as a health professional can. And you will often have a choice in how to make these adjustments. For example, some people may choose to take more insulin or alter their medication to cover a particular meal or period of stress. Others may choose to exercise more. A lot of variations are possible. There isn't an absolute, rigid, you-must-live-this-way diabetes control program for anybody. We feel these choices should be left up to you, the patient. But you can't make these choices intelligently unless you're taught how. And you *can* be taught. Certainly if physicians can learn it and I can learn it and the health-care team I work with can learn it, you can learn it too.

We've learned it because we practice, but mostly we've learned it because our patients have taught us. We take our patients' records and examine them and have the patients tell us what happened. Then, when we've done this often enough, we come up with some guidelines.

For example, we may say, "Gee, it looks like every time somebody has had pan pizza, their blood sugars are much higher than when they eat thin-crust pizza. There must be a pattern here." You can do this kind of analysis on yourself. You can also see, using your blood sugar tests, the different effects of exercise and medication. It's really not a terribly difficult decision-making process. The important part of it is learning to be creative and flexible and to realize that there's more than one way to skin a cat.

JUNE AND BARBARA: You mentioned in your introduction that you managed your diabetes with diet for eight years and now you're on oral hypoglycemic agents—or, as most of us call them, the pills. Why did you add this kind of medication to your therapy and what are these pills, anyway?

VIRGINIA: These are the class of drugs called sulfonylureas (pronounced sul-faw-nul-u-re-us. It took me two years to learn how to say this. That's why most of us just call them "pills.") These medications are specifically for the treatment of Type II diabetes. They have two different kinds of actions. One is the pancreatic effect. This means they increase your level of insulin by kicking your pancreas to produce a little more. But if you're insulin deficient, there's nothing there to kick out. It's like kicking a dead horse. That's why these pills are only useful for people who have Type II diabetes and are still making insulin.

The second effect of these pills is to make you more receptive to your own insulin at the cell receptor level. It is not known which of these two mechanisms provides the most benefit. These drugs have been on the market for 35 years, but the current drugs most commonly used are the second generation, which came out in the early '80s. There are two main second-generation oral agents: glyburide and glypizide.

JUNE AND BARBARA: Could you explain these so that people who take them or will be taking them understand how they work?

VIRGINIA: The brand names for glyburide are Micronase, Glynase, and Diabeta. This group has a maximum daily dose of 12 to 20 mg (milligrams). They are very effective. Theoretically they could be taken once a day, but we have noticed that splitting the daily dose, taking half before breakfast and half before supper, provides a better effect since Type II diabetics primarily have a problem with fasting blood sugar. If that's your problem, you should try splitting your medication.

Glypizide is better known by the brand name Glucotrol. The maximum daily dose is 40 mg and it is also a very effective oral agent. It has a shorter life than glyburide so most people take it every 12 hours. Glypizide is probably the safer drug for an older person since there is less chance of it causing hypoglycemia.

JUNE AND BARBARA: How does the second generation of pills differ from the first?

VIRGINIA: They're just a more potent form of the first generation. In other words, you can take less of the drug and therefore have fewer side effects. Not many drugs for diseases that affect as many people as diabetes does are basically the same ones that have been in use for 35 years.

When you think about technology and all the new things we have available to treat different diseases, it's funny that we should still be using these 35-year-old medications—which, incidentally, were discovered by accident during research on sulfa antibiotics during World War II. When it was discovered that this group of drugs caused hypoglycemia in patients, doctors started to make use of this hypoglycemic effect to treat Type II diabetes.

In the '60s, some researchers developed the theory that these drugs could increase the risk of heart disease, and as a result they went out of favor for a while. In recent years, however, that research has been refuted by other studies and now they are generally felt to be very safe drugs. One exception is during pregnancy. These drugs may cause birth defects, and women who have even a remote chance of becoming pregnant should not be taking these medications.

JUNE AND BARBARA: Why do you think that theory of the cardiovascular risk of pills got started?

VIRGINIA: Probably because the pills created a higher level of insulin in the body and that was what caused the cardiovascular problems. Now that we know more about Type II diabetes, we realize that it is the high insulin level that predisposes people with the disease to increased risk of cardiovascular problems. It doesn't make any difference if their insulin level is high because their extreme insulin resistance is causing their own bodies to pump out extra insulin, or because they are put on oral hypoglycemics that kick their pancreases to make more insulin, or because they take insulin by injection. It's the increased insulin level, not how it got there, that increases the cardiovascular risk. In fact, if diabetes were given credit for all of the cardiovascular deaths and disabilities that it causes, it would be rated much higher as a national concern than it currently is.

JUNE AND BARBARA: What are the positive benefits of the pills?

VIRGINIA: Many people can control their diabetes very successfully on the oral agents, even after they flunk out on diet alone. As you mentioned, at first I was able to control my diabetes with diet and was perking along just fine, always keeping my fasting blood sugar under 130 and my glycohemoglobin within the normal range. Then I distinctly remember getting a bad cold with bronchitis. I was very sick, with the kind of laid-up-for-a-week illness that I almost never get. My fasting blood sugar popped up to 180, and it stayed that way even after I got well. I tried many different things to bring my blood sugar down, including changing my diet. But no matter what I did, I just couldn't consistently stay in control for any length of time. After several months of this I decided to start on an oral agent. The one that I took, glyburide, worked fairly well to control my blood sugars although they still weren't nearly the level that I wanted.

Finally I figured out that exercise and a low-fat diet might be the therapy I needed. Following this regimen I lost 16 pounds and gained good diabetes control. I now know from this personal experience and from my work with patients that there is no escaping the need for exercise and diet along with the pills or insulin or both. Insulin and pills are not what you do instead of diet and exercise, they're just part of the armamentarium. Diet and exercise are still the key factors in managing Type II diabetes.

JUNE AND BARBARA: Are you still taking the pills?

VIRGINIA: I'm still taking them, but only rarely. If my blood sugars are up, I'll take a couple.

JUNE AND BARBARA: You can't just pop them now and then, can you? Isn't that kind of risky?

VIRGINIA: Actually, they're very safe drugs. The most common side effect of these oral agents is hypoglycemia, and that's pretty rare. Your doctor or nurse can teach you how to use the pills intermittently. Not everybody needs to go on them and stay on them forever. You should use blood glucose monitoring and adjust your dose of the oral agents just as people adjust their doses of insulin.

JUNE AND BARBARA: Is there any final warning about using the pills?

VIRGINIA: Although, as I said, they are very safe, there are a couple of things to keep in mind. If you're using chloropramide, a first-generation drug known as Diabenese, if you drink an alcoholic beverage you can get a bright red flushing of the skin—an alcohol flush. On any of the drugs you do have to make sure that your liver and kidney functions are up to speed. Otherwise the body won't be able to excrete them effectively.

JUNE AND BARBARA: If you're allergic to sulfa antibiotics, will you also be allergic to their relatives, the sulfonylureas?

VIRGINIA: Not necessarily. Many times we have patients tell us they're allergic to sulfa drugs but they've been on an oral agent for many years with no problems. Rarely is a person who is allergic to sulfa antibiotics also allergic to the sulfonylureas. If you're the kind of person who has had extremely dramatic symptoms or reactions to a sulfa drug—for example, difficulty in breathing—you should talk this over with your physician before you use one of these medications. He or she can monitor you and make decisions about whether this is the right drug for you. At least be aware of possible adverse reactions and be ready to treat any allergic response that you might have, unlikely though it may be.

JUNE AND BARBARA: We've heard of some people taking both pills and insulin. Under what circumstances is that combination used?

VIRGINIA: If you're on the maximum oral agent dose and your fasting blood sugar is still too high—and therefore your blood sugar will be too high for the rest of the day (as the fasting goes, so goes the rest of the day)—some physicians will add NPH (slow-acting) insulin at bedtime. By adding this dose of NPH, you can often normalize the fasting blood sugar. The pills will then work fine for the rest of the day. We call this BIDS: bedtime insulin, daytime sulfonylureas. It provides a nice alternative to having to go totally onto insulin. Also in selected individuals we use the pills and insulin in combination to avoid going to much higher doses of insulin which could predispose the person to weight gain.

JUNE AND BARBARA: Aren't there any newer, better pills available—or about to be available—that might allow more people to stay off insulin longer?

VIRGINIA: As you can infer from all that I've said, what we really need is a drug that will correct that Type II-R problem of insulin resistance. And, fortunately, there are drugs in the research pipeline right now that will improve the receptors' utilization of insulin. With these your insulin level will drop, which will allow you to lose weight. I personally can't wait until they're on the market. Unfortunately, it could be quite a few more years before we see them on the market. Until the happy day of their arrival, we'll just have to continue working with what we have in the drug line and working on lifestyle changes to improve our conditions.

A more important reason to work diligently on keeping your blood sugars under control is that you don't want your body to be damaged. You want to stay in good shape so you can benefit from the new drugs when they arrive. One thing to note about the second generation of drugs, the ones that are currently in use, is that they are getting ready to go off of patent in 1993. In other words, generic forms of these drugs will show up on the market, and the prices will come down. And that's always good news!

JUNE AND BARBARA: Who makes the decision that a person should go on insulin and how is this determined?

VIRGINIA: Even though Type II diabetes is also called non-insulin-dependent diabetes, it's very common for Type II's to go on insulin. This makes for a lot of confusion, because as many as 25 to 50 percent of Type II's will eventually be using insulin to manage their diabetes. How is this determined? Typically people with Type II diabetes, when diagnosed, can get along with diet and exercise. Then when their insulin production deficit becomes so large that they cannot overcome their resistance, they're given the oral agents. As we've said, the pills stimulate people's own insulin-making capability, plus they cause them to use their own insulin a little better. That works for a while. The average time that oral agents work is between five and seven years, although it can be much less time or longer. I have a patient who has been on pills for 25 years. Granted, he's the only one I've seen who has made use of them that long. It's very unusual, but possible.

Now let's say that you've exhausted all efforts with diet and exercise and the oral agents are no longer controlling your blood sugar in the range that you and your physician have determined to be appropriate. Probably your fasting blood sugars are significantly over 150 and after-meal blood sugars are significantly over 200. So you are told that you should go on insulin.

JUNE AND BARBARA: What happens next? How do you "go on insulin"? What kind of insulin and how much?

VIRGINIA: There are several different ways. Some physicians will simply take you off all oral agents and start you on an insulin regimen. Others in recent years have found that if they can just get the fasting blood sugar normal, then the rest of the day will be controlled just fine with pills. They may start you on one injection of NPH insulin at bedtime. NPH insulin is slow acting and has its peak action about eight hours after injection. The idea is that it will lower your blood sugar just about the time in the early morning hours that it ordinarily starts to go up because of excessive liver glucose production. This program, as I've mentioned, is called BIDS, bedtime insulin, daytime sulfonylureas.

If you fail on the pills, your physician may decide not to use pills at all anymore, but to go exclusively to insulin. Unit for unit, insulin is much cheaper than pills. If you're going to have to go on insulin anyway, some doctors reason, why not go straight to insulin to begin with and use insulin only? In that case, the 70/30 premixed insulin is ideal for Type II diabetics. This means that in any dose that you draw up, 70 percent of the units will be NPH-type insulin (slow acting) and 30 percent will be Regular insulin (fast acting). I favor this system myself, because it makes more sense for Type II's. Remember, one of the three errors in metabolism that Type II's have is abnormal insulin production. In other words, you don't get a first-phase insulin response. So when you eat a meal, you don't get that insulin right away to keep your blood sugar from soaring after the meal. That's why you need to have Regular (fast-acting) insulin before breakfast, just like a Type I diabetic, and then NPH in the middle of the day to cover lunch. Notice, though, in Figure 2.1 that the NPH starts running out during dinner; that's the main reason most patients go on two shots a day of 70/30 insulin. This can be very convenient: just an injection before breakfast and before supper. It provides excellent coverage for most Type II's.

Figure 2.1 Timing of Insulin Action

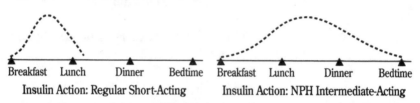

Insulin Action: Regular Short-Acting   Insulin Action: NPH Intermediate-Acting

On the 70/30 twice-a-day regime you'll need more insulin in the evening than in the morning. This is because your insulin resistance causes excessive liver glucose during the night. I tell my patients that we can't be shy about using however much insulin it takes. The most important key for control in the Type II-R on insulin is to use however much insulin it takes to get those blood sugars down. If you start out with a normal fasting blood sugar, it will take a lot less insulin to manage it throughout the day.

Another common regimen uses NPH and Regular insulin that the patient mixes himself or herself. This is especially appropriate for Type II-D's, because they do not have that cushion of insulin to keep their blood sugars relatively stable. NPH plus Regular is used before breakfast, Regular and NPH before supper, or Regular alone before supper and NPH at bedtime. Doing this allows you to adjust the Regular insulin doses based on your blood sugar level at the time and depending on what you plan to eat at breakfast and supper. This adds a certain level of flexibility.

Yet another variation is to use Regular insulin before each meal and not take any NPH until bedtime. This is the "treat only the problem" approach. Because some Type II-R's have enough of their own insulin for basal coverage (baseline metabolism when not eating), they could have good blood glucose levels if they never ate (not a good long-term solution). If they take Regular before each meal and NPH before bed (some physicians use

Lente before bed), they're using insulin to supplement the problem areas during the day.

JUNE AND BARBARA: We notice that you've abandoned the old system of putting all Type II's on just one shot of NPH every morning. That was certainly an easy way to go, and it was June's regime for years until she wised up and suggested to her doctor that she would like to use Regular before each meal. Is the one-shot-a-day system ever used today?

VIRGINIA: Yes, all too often Type II's are put on only one shot a day. Almost always they should be taking more than one shot, and it should not be NPH alone. Let me explain why. NPH, as we noted, has a slow onset. It doesn't even start working for an hour or two, then it peaks in 8 to 10 hours and is usually gone in about 14 hours. In other words, it doesn't last all 24 hours. If you take one shot in the morning of NPH, your blood sugar is going to go real high after breakfast, then a peak of NPH in the afternoon will pull you back down. That's not a good way to go. It lets the blood sugar fluctuate too widely during the day. It just doesn't feel good for our blood sugar to swing a hundred points. Mother Nature did not design us that way. We were designed to have a blood sugar fluctuation of no more than 30–40 points throughout the day. If we can mimic that for people with diabetes, they feel better.

JUNE AND BARBARA: There are so many kinds of insulin on the market now that a beginner might be very confused when trying to buy the particular one their doctor has prescribed. When June started using insulin 25 years ago, there were few choices, because we had only animal insulins (made from the pancreases of pigs or cattle). Now, of course, in addition to animal insulins we have the human insulins, which are exactly like the insulin the body makes. (Manufactured human insulin is made with recombinant DNA genetic engineering techniques.) Isn't it hard to explain all this to new insulin takers?

VIRGINIA: It's not really as complicated as it sounds at first. Only two companies in the United States make insulin: Eli Lilly and Novo Nordisk. And there are only four major types with different speeds of action.

1. Regular is the short-acting kind that starts working in about 45 minutes and peaks (has its strongest effect) in 2 or 3 hours and is gone in 4 or 5 hours.

2. The intermediate-acting insulins are NPH, by far the most commonly used, and Lente. (NPH stands for neutral protamine of Hagedorn. Dr. Hagedorn of Denmark invented this insulin and named it after himself.) NPH starts to work in 30 to 90 minutes, peaks between 6 and 8 hours, and lasts about 12 hours.

3. The only long-acting insulin is Ultralente. The human kind has an onset of 1 to 3 hours, a peak that can span 8 to 14 hours, and lasts 18 to 24 hours. The Ultralente from animal sources has a delayed onset of 4 to 6 hours, a peak that can span 8 to 16 hours, and a duration of 25 to 36 hours.

4. There are several premixed combinations of NPH and Regular. There is the combination of 70 percent NPH and 30 percent Regular, which we favor in New Mexico for our Type II-R's. And now a 50/50 mix is available. In Europe 60/40, 80/20, and 90/10 mixes are available. (Those Europeans must be pretty lazy if they don't ever want to be bothered mixing their own insulin dosage.)

As far as I'm concerned, cows should get beef insulin, pigs should get pork insulin, and people should get human insulin. I believe pharmacies could quit carrying all those formulations of animal insulin. I guess some people still take them just because they have never bothered to ask their doctor about switching. Why should you take human insulin? Because it's the insulin your body would make if it could. It is less likely to cause your body to make antibodies. When your body is making antibodies to the foreign protein in pork insulin or the three foreign proteins in beef insulin, then it is diminishing the effect of the insulin injection and possibly causing erratic action of that insulin.

Incidentally, there used to be another long-lasting insulin like Ultralente called PZI (protamine zinc insulin). It went off the market two years ago, but this didn't make the front pages of newspapers, because the only ones who missed it were cats with diabetes. It seems that veterinarians had found it to be the preferred insulin for diabetic cats. I'm sure vets have found a suitable alternative.

JUNE AND BARBARA: Doesn't taking insulin cause diabetics to gain weight? You've told us that it's a powerful fat-generating hormone.

VIRGINIA: Yes, it very well could. The person with Type II diabetes probably has enough insulin on board but is very resistant to it. Now we add more with injections. If you think about it, if your blood sugar has been running 250 and your weight has been staying stable, it figures that a fair amount of your calories have been going out in the toilet, because the extra sugar in the blood stream is being spilled into the urine. If we give you enough insulin to get your blood sugar down to normal, those calories that were putting sugar into your urine have to go somewhere else, right? Probably right to your thighs.

JUNE AND BARBARA: If this is so, how can you avoid gaining weight?

VIRGINIA: When you start insulin, you just have to give up one thing: give up some fat in your diet. Cut out something that will be equivalent to a few hundred calories a day. That could be the mayonnaise on your sandwich at lunch, the dressing on your salad, or the butter on your bread. It won't be something you'd miss a whole bunch, but you must give up some calories to keep your weight from going up.

JUNE AND BARBARA: What's the best way to teach people how to inject insulin? Do you still use an orange to practice with?

VIRGINIA: Absolutely not! What a waste of a perfectly good orange. When a patient who has to go on insulin comes to me to learn how to inject, I don't talk about anything else, I just get straight to the injection procedure. I have them give themselves an injection using sterile water, so they can find out that it's not a real big deal. It doesn't hurt if you do it right. Once they've done their first injection, then we can talk about other things such as managing their blood sugars.

So many people have such an exaggerated fear of shots and needles that we've had to come up with innovative ways to get them through that barrier (see page 147). One thing I've discovered for people with severe needle phobia is never to use an alcohol swab to prepare for the injection. The smell of alcohol sends them back to being five years old and being chased around the doctor's office by a nurse who had to hold them down to give them a shot. So no alcohol swab. Just draw up the sterile water and inject immediately. Then they can relax because they know it's nothing. They've been worried so long, now at last they're relieved.

Using alcohol on your skin is really an unnecessary waste of money and cotton and alcohol. We tell people that the little germs on your skin have been buddies with your body for years, and nobody ever gets an infection from themselves. Lots of studies have been done on this. A study was even done of diabetic kids at camp. Can you imagine how dirty kids get? And none of them ever got an infection from their insulin shots. Another tip: you can reuse your insulin syringes. The label on a syringe says that you should use it once and then destroy it, but that's for hospitals, since needles are never shared between patients. When I recommend to patients that they reuse their syringes, they'll ask, "How many times?" My answer is that you'll know. When it bounces off your tummy, it's time to quit using that one. Most people find that after four or five times, they should switch to a new syringe.

JUNE AND BARBARA: We knew one man who always used his syringes around 24 times. He said he actually liked them better when they got dull! We also knew an environmentally concerned woman who searched in vain everywhere for one of those old glass syringes with detachable needles. She didn't want to load the landfill with disposable syringes. She finally had to compromise by using her syringes over and over again.

We consider disposable syringes to be one of the greatest improvements in diabetes injection ease. Are there any even newer ways to make insulin injecting, if not pleasant, at least more convenient?

VIRGINIA: Yes, there are many new ways to make your life much easier as far as insulin injections are concerned. There is a device called the Novolin™ pen that holds the insulin and you just dial the dose. The newest product is the Novolin Prefilled™ Syringe, which comes preloaded with 150 units of Novolin™ 70/30 human insulin. It's about the size of a pen and you use the "cap" to set a dose of up to 58 units. It delivers when you inject the needle and press the pushbutton at the end. When it's empty you dispose of it like a regular syringe. People love its simplicity, convenience, and accuracy. We have many people on pen devices, and I feel every patient should be offered a choice of insulin delivery systems.

JUNE AND BARBARA: Some Type II-D's (and possibly even some II-R's) may be interested in the insulin infusion pumps that are advertised as the best way to get good control. We know a lot of people who gained total happiness using a pump. What's your opinion of the pump system?

VIRGINIA: Pumps use what we call the basal-bolus insulin program. Basal refers to the insulin coverage needed to maintain blood glucose levels at times other than at meals. The bolus insulin (a concentrated dose) is used to cover meals. This schedule is designed to imitate the way your body handles its insulin output (a little bit all the time and more before meals). You don't have to be on a pump to use this system. You can use injections of Ultralente insulin morning and evening for a very nice basal effect and injections of Regular insulin before each meal. This gives you a lot more flexibility in being able to change your schedule, and being able to eat more or less at different meals. You can also exercise without having an insulin peak sneak up on you. We've had a lot of success with this program. Some people call it "the poor man's pump," because syringes cost a lot less than pumps.

The cost of pumps is the reason everybody on insulin doesn't use them. It costs around $4,000 to get started on a pump. For people who are very difficult to control, pumps are certainly a wonderful option, but most people who can manage their diabetes with exercise, oral agents, or injections see the pump as an unnecessary expense and more trouble to maintain than it's worth.

By way of example, I have one patient who is a Type II diabetic on a pump. She has had tremendous problems controlling her blood sugar for many years. She can take neither NPH nor Lente insulins because of allergies. She could tolerate Regular but didn't like taking injections five or six times a day. She finally came to me and said, "I want a pump." On the pump her control was greatly improved. She enjoyed the ability to eat less at some times and more at other meals. She appreciated this new flexibility and ease of use.

She is a child psychologist, easily the best one I've ever met. When she got her pump and started it up, she noticed it made a clicking sound. With every little basal dose it gave, it clicked. She asked how to turn off the clicks. I told her she couldn't because that's how she knew the pump was working. She said, "The kids will go nuts over this. They're going to hate it and it's going to be distracting. This is going to be a big problem in my practice." She put the device inside an oven mitt and anything else she could find to muffle the sound. Then she started telling her young clients that she was a bionic woman and her body made clicks. They had no problem at all understanding that. It was only the parents who found her distracting. They were the ones glancing around the room with funny looks on their faces when they heard her click. By the way, she is now on a new pump, the Disetronic, that doesn't click, and she really loves it!

JUNE AND BARBARA: People who saw the movie *Reversal of Fortune* know that the contention of the prosecution was that Klaus von Bulow gave his wife a huge dose of insulin to kill her. She did not die but is in what appears to be an endless coma. Some moviegoers might have gotten the idea that insulin is a lethal drug or even a murder weapon. What are the real dangers, if any, of taking insulin and how do you set people's minds at ease on this score?

VIRGINIA: If you saw the movie, then you know what a bad idea it is to try to kill somebody with insulin. Granted that Sunny von

Bulow is a vegetable today, but with normal doses of insulin the body has tremendous protective mechanisms to prevent problems from hypoglycemia. If your blood sugar starts getting too low, the pancreas starts increasing production of glucagon (the hormone that causes an increase in blood sugar; in other words, it has the opposite function of insulin). The glucagon tells the liver to start pouring glucose out. Eventually the body will even start breaking down muscle and fat to make sure there is enough fuel available.

Under ordinary circumstances, even when a person's blood sugar drops so low that they pass out, which is rare and virtually nonexistent in Type II-R's (though it could happen with Type I's or Type II-D's), the body uses counterregulatory hormones such as epinephrine to generate enough glucose to protect the body and especially the brain. These mechanisms provide enough glucose to revive you. With the massive doses of insulin that Sunny von Bulow received, her brain was allowed to go without fuel long enough to be damaged.

Unlike in Type I diabetes, Type II-R's have such a huge level of stored glucose in the liver that they rarely experience any hypoglycemia, let alone pass out from low blood sugar. It is possible, though, to experience the feelings of hypoglycemia, even at a higher than normal level of blood glucose, if the brain has become what we call "glucose intoxicated." This means that if you are used to running blood sugars of 300 or 400 points and we quickly bring your blood sugar down to 150 or less, you may experience the symptoms of true hypoglycemia—for example, feeling shaky, sweaty, irritable, headachy. This happens even though your blood sugar is at or near a normal level.

If this happens to you, eat a small snack such as a few crackers. Then with a little rest, the feeling will go away. We want to avoid overtreating that pseudohypoglycemia, because what will happen is that you'll just get your blood sugar back up to 300 and you'll never adapt to normal blood sugars. If you're used to running high blood sugars, you will usually adapt to normal ones in a couple of weeks. Then you'll feel better in the long run.

JUNE AND BARBARA: We've had many people come to us with the complaint that they suffer from hypoglycemia—the disease, not the hypoglycemic episodes that insulin-dependent diabetics sometimes experience. They're looking for books that might help them overcome the awful feelings of nervousness and depression that hypoglycemia causes. We don't know of any really good book for hypoglycemics, but we do warn them that we've heard this condition can be a precursor of diabetes. What we want to know is how is it possible to go from having a low blood sugar condition to the very reverse?

VIRGINIA: To understand that, all you have to do is remember that many, many years before being diagnosed with diabetes, the Type II diabetic lost the first-phase insulin response. If you don't have that first-phase insulin response, then when you eat a meal that is especially high in simple carbohydrates, you're going to get a real quick rise in blood glucose. This will stimulate an even bigger second-stage insulin response that in two to three hours will cause you to be hypoglycemic. We call this reactive hypoglycemia. This is the explanation of why many people tell you that they were "hypoglycemic" for years and then eventually turned into Type II diabetics, even though they seem like opposite conditions. Reactive hypoglycemia, in other words, can be one stage in the evolution of Type II diabetes.

I have patients who say that every time they eat a candy bar or drink a Coke they feel sick. There is a simple solution to this problem: just don't do it! The diet for the person with reactive hypoglycemia is the same as for the person with diabetes. That is, eat foods high in fiber, low in sugar, low in fat—in other words, a good healthy diet. And don't ever drink liquid sugar—meaning soft drinks or fruit juice.

JUNE AND BARBARA: Is insulin a prescription drug in New Mexico? In California you don't need a prescription. How about other states?

VIRGINIA: Insulin is available without prescription everywhere in the United States. This is so it will be available in case of an emergency need by a person with diabetes. Some states though, regulate the purchase of syringes and require a prescription for a syringe.

If you're going to be traveling, it's important that you carry your insulin with you and not check it with your luggage. But if you ever lose your insulin or run out of it, you can always get more. This is why it's important to carry a prescription or the name of your insulin so you'll know exactly what kind to buy. I always advise people who are first starting on insulin to tear off the box top and put it in their purse or billfold. That way they will know the brand name and type of insulin in case they're ever out of their home area and have to buy it.

Fortunately, in this country insulin is extremely inexpensive. This is rather surprising when you think about all the technology that goes into human insulin production using the DNA technique. Researchers have trained little bacteria or yeast to pump out the chains of amino acids that make up human insulin. (Come to think of it, though, they don't even pay these little workers minimum wage.) The insulin is as pure as it can get and it only costs $12 to $20 a bottle, which lasts most people three to four weeks. It is one of the cheapest prescriptions today.

JUNE AND BARBARA: If you want to do yourself in financially, just buy a bottle of insulin in Europe. In Switzerland it was going for $34 a bottle in 1992. And since foreign brands have different manufacturers and names for the various types of insulin, you can really get yourself in a bind if you leave home without enough extra bottles to see you through any emergency.

Unexpected things happen when you're out of your routine and in far-off places. June once left her insulin on the seat of the airplane when arriving in Hawaii. Fortunately she called the airport and they held it for her even though she was silly enough not to have her name on the case in which she was carrying it. Another time her Regular insulin clouded up in France (the clouding was caused by silicon from repeated needle insertions into the bottle and was harmless, but she didn't know that). Then we had the experience of buying an insulin of a different strength (U40 instead of U100) and having to do complex calculations to get the correct dosage. Let her foolishness be a lesson to you (though most insulins are now the same strength abroad as here).

Since many diabetes supplies—insulin, pills, test strips—have expiration dates, how many weeks' or months' supply should a person buy? You don't want to run out, but you also don't want to let expensive products expire. There must be some way to be safe but not sorry when you look in your medicine chest.

VIRGINIA: When insulin is manufactured, a two-year expiration date is marked on the bottle. So the farthest out you can get insulin is a two-year expiration date, but one-year expiration from the time you purchase it should be more than adequate. You probably only need to keep a month's supply. Since the insulin you purchase from the drugstore has been carefully refrigerated, you'll want to keep your spare bottles in the refrigerator, too. (The insert in the Novo Nordisk insulins says, "Insulin should be stored in a cold place, preferably in a refrigerator.") The insulin you are currently using can be kept at room temperature and it can be kept for a month that way. If you're one of those people who don't use up a bottle in a month, I would suggest keeping it in the fridge and taking it out about an hour before you're going to use it. If you use it up in two or three weeks, leaving it at room temperature is no problem. (By the way, the inside of your car is not considered room temperature.)

Most syringes have an expiration date, but as long as they haven't been contaminated they're probably just fine.

JUNE AND BARBARA: What do you mean by contaminated? We've never heard of that.

VIRGINIA: Let's say you found them in the garage in storage and you see that years ago they got wet and have been chewed on by mice. Those syringes you'd want to dispose of. If they're still in their plastic bag or wrapper and have not had their protective covers removed and have not been through an atomic bomb attack, they should be OK.

JUNE AND BARBARA: So far June's syringes have survived a number of California earthquakes. But unlike syringes, pills can get out of date, can't they?

VIRGINIA: Yes, oral agents usually have an expiration date but that date is usually several years out, so that's no problem. The real problem with stocking up on any medication too far ahead is that if for some reason your physician should decide that you need to change the medication regimen, you're stuck with these drugs; you can't take them back. Could you use oral agents beyond the expiration date? Probably, but the pharmacists won't tell you that it's OK. I would talk to my doctor about this. I will tell you, though, that I teach a class in a nursing school where some of my students are in the military. They tell me that the military uses drugs past their expiration date. This is one of the ways they save money. There seems to be no problem with the "expired" drugs.

JUNE AND BARBARA: How about test strips? Sometimes people buy a lot of them at once to get a better price and then they find them going out of date.

VIRGINIA: Test strips are the one item to be careful with. They do go bad. I would watch the expiration date and I would not buy any strips whose date is not at least six months away. Granted, you would probably use them up before a slightly earlier expiration date, but it's best to be on the safe side. Strips are very fragile, very sensitive to moisture or excessive heat. If left in the heat or the cold, in the car, or with the lid off the bottle—especially in the damp atmosphere of a bathroom—they can be damaged.

JUNE AND BARBARA: *Diabetes Forecast* publishes a "Buyer's Guide to Diabetes Products" each year in its October issue. It's an extremely detailed listing and description of all products of all kinds, from carrying cases to insulin pumps to medical IDs. At the end is a complete list of manufacturers and suppliers with their addresses and 800 numbers. How helpful do you find this information, and what's the best way to use it?

VIRGINIA: The problem with this information is that there is no evaluation of the products. They list junk meters right up there equally with the quality meters. Therefore, there is no way to compare the products. Do I find this guide helpful? Not really. I already know the manufacturers' 800 numbers, but I guess for some people this may be a place to call and ask questions. I wish *Consumer Reports* would do an article giving a qualitative analysis of the different meters. Short of waiting for that to happen, you can always ask your diabetes educator. Your diabetes educator has probably had more experience with all of these products than any other single person and can help you decide on the best product for you.

JUNE AND BARBARA: What do you think of mail-order sources for purchasing supplies and equipment? About 10 different ones in different states advertise each month in the "Shopper's Guide" section at the back of *Diabetes Forecast*. Others send out catalogs and newsletters. Have many of your patients used these services and found them advantageous?

VIRGINIA: Some people do like them, because they don't have to drive around town to find things. Having supplies delivered right to your door saves time. But often the prices of the mail-order supplies are very similar to the prices at the discount houses in your town, and buying locally saves you the cost of shipping, handling, and delivery (although if you're dealing with an out-of-state mail-order house, you can save the sales tax). I'd say it's a toss-up. Some people like mail-order sources and others don't find them to be advantageous.

CHAPTER 3

EXERCISE:
YOUR LIFETIME
SAVING PLAN

Personal finance expert Jane Bryant Quinn, in her book *Making the Most of Your Money,* advises that for lifetime financial security you should always "Pay yourself first." By this she means that out of whatever dollars you make each month you should set aside 10 percent for saving before you do anything else with your money. Our advice for exercise is the same as hers for money. Before you plan anything else in your day, set aside 10 percent of your available time—for most of us that will average out at from 30 to 90 minutes—for exercise. Ms. Quinn is adamant that financial investment should be regular and inviolable; you should never say, "There's something I'd rather do with my money right now. I'll skip saving this month and double the amount next month." And we're adamant that exercise should be regular and inviolable; you should never say, "There's something I'd rather do with my time today. I'll skip my exercise and do twice as much tomorrow." The reason for both rules is that the saving and the exercise have to be a routine, a habit, and if you break the routine once it's easier to break it the next time . . . and the next . . . and the next, until you wake up one morning and find yourself in deep financial or physical trouble.

Ms. Quinn advocates different kinds of investments for different people. Some people aren't comfortable with the gyrations of the stock market and prefer mutual funds or the even more secure and stable money market accounts and T-bills. Some don't like the trouble of handling rental property, while others are willing to expend effort on property management in exchange for income and tax advantages. She even suggests a variety of investments for the same person to create a balanced saving portfolio and to avoid the risk of putting all your financial eggs in one basket.

We feel the same way about exercise. Some people like to play tennis, some enjoy square dancing, hiking, skating, walking, swimming, skiing, and, although most people don't or can't invest the time and effort it takes to run marathons, there are those who believe it's worth all the tremendous exertion in exchange for the mind and body benefits they derive from marathons. We also think that a balanced exercise portfolio is a good idea. Combining something that's aerobic with some strength training and possibly a competitive sport will give you activities to see you through all weather, seasonal, and personal mood fluctuations and will condition all parts of your body.

It's not easy to adhere to your savings program when you see others blowing their money on clothes or cars or vacations whenever they feel like it, with not a thought in the world for their economic futures. And it's not easy to stick to your exercise program when you're awash in a sea of workaholics who grind away 14 hours a day and couch potatoes whose major exercise is reaching for a bowl of potato chips or punching buttons on the TV remote.

But the rewards are there for both Ms. Quinn's plan and ours. If you religiously follow her counsel, it's amazing the wealth you will be able to accumulate in a lifetime. You will be financially comfortable and secure when others about you are desperately floating loans or filing for bankruptcy or moving in with relatives. If you

religiously follow our counsel, it's amazing the health
you will be able to enjoy for your lifetime. You will be
youthfully vigorous and vital when your contemporaries
are sluggish and bloated and old before their time. On
top of that, our plan has a big dividend, one that's as
good in terms of your health as winning the lottery
would be in terms of your wealth: *your diabetes will be
in good control.*

And here's the best part: both these plans—the saving and the exercise—that are so beneficial for your
well-being, can evolve into a joy and a pleasure if you
enter into the spirit and make a challenging game of
them.

We'll leave it up to Ms. Quinn and others to put you
on the road to a lifetime money saving program. We're
here to put you on the road to a lifetime health saving
program and help you put your best foot forward.

—June and Barbara

What You'll Find in This Chapter

Benefits of Exercise
Setting Goals
Aerobics
Walking; Shoes and Socks
Strength Training

BARBARA AND JUNE: Virginia, you must be aware that both of
us are exercise fanatics. We'll bet, though, that you didn't know
we've written three entire books about sports—one on downhill
skiing, one on cross-country skiing, and one on bicycling. And in
1977, with the help of 158 exercise enthusiasts who have diabetes,
we published the first book ever to deal solely with exercise therapy for diabetes: *The Diabetic's Sports and Exercise Book; How to
Play Your Way to Better Health.* Unfortunately it is out of print, but
we still get calls for it because nothing more extensive has ever
come out to replace it.

We still feel just as passionately about the value of exercise for
people with diabetes as we did then. And more than ever we keep

preaching that others should become as fanatic about exercise as we are. Now that we've revealed our prejudice up front, we'll ask you how you rank exercise as a part of diabetes treatment.

VIRGINIA: Probably when the whole truth is known, it will turn out that exercise is everything. But, frankly, it's the hardest thing for me to get a grip on. I know that when we find the gene for Type II diabetes, he will be stretched out on his back with his feet up! I've not met one Type II-R who *loves* to exercise. It's a constant battle for us to get out and hoof it down the road even though it's the most important part of keeping diabetes in control.

Once again, I go back to the idea of living like our ancestors: being very physically active and eating a low-fat, high-fiber diet. The diet is much easier for me to master than the exercise. I constantly battle with myself to get out there and get moving. When other people talk about how good exercise feels, I wonder if there's some genetic reason that we Type II-R's don't get addicted to it. Is it related to the fact that we don't use glucose the same way "normal" people do?

JUNE AND BARBARA: We can see, Virginia, that you're dragging your feet on exercise even while recognizing and acknowledging its crucial importance. So why don't we trade places in this chapter? We'll try to be so convincing about exercise that you'll find yourself skipping out the door with breathless anticipation.

VIRGINIA: I jump at the chance to accept your offer. Or, considering my feelings about exercise, maybe I'll just go stretch out on my back with my feet up and listen to your every word. Go ahead, convert me.

JUNE AND BARBARA: First, we want to make a little philosophical statement. We think every nurse and doctor—and every person with diabetes—should cease calling exercise a prescription, as in the question, "What is your exercise prescription?" or "This is your exercise prescription for the first month." Don't ever think of exercise as a prescription, some kind of bitter pill to swallow for your own good. Think of it as an opportunity to have fun, to go out and play the way you did as a kid.

Now, having put you in the right frame of mind, we can show you what exercise can do for you and how to get yourself doing it.

VIRGINIA: All right, what *can* exercise do for me? (I'm afraid I already know the answer to this!)

JUNE AND BARBARA: We know you know all the merits of exercise for people with diabetes, but in a sense you don't. As one of Leo Buscaglia's wisest teachers said to him: "To know and not to do is not to know." Maybe it's like taking skiing or tennis lessons. You hear the same thing over and over from different instructors until one day something clicks and you finally really get it. So here we go.

Exercise makes everything about diabetes therapy easier. It makes it easier to:

- control your blood sugar
- lose weight
- keep fit in the cardiovascular sense
- lower your blood fats
- increase your muscle strength and flexibility
- deter the "inevitable" process of aging
- avoid complications
- keep your spirits high and enhance your appearance and self-esteem

VIRGINIA: As a health professional, I concur with your entire list. I might add that the most important thing exercise does for overweight Type II-R's is to change their metabolism so that they burn more calories even if they're sitting still. The books that explain this phenomenon best are those by Covert Bailey, who first published his *Fit or Fat?* in 1977 and since then *The New Fit or Fat?* as well as *Fit-or-Fat Target Diet, Fit-or-Fat Recipes,* and *Fit-or-Fat Woman.* What he says, over and over again, is that "the ultimate cure for obesity is exercise."

JUNE AND BARBARA: Yes, we've been preaching the Covert Bailey gospel since he came out with his first book. What people loved about his program was that initially he recommended a total of only 12 minutes of continuous aerobic exercise three times a week. That's not much time to give up for so much in return. Have you had any patients who have used the Covert Bailey program and found it helped them lose weight and significantly improve their diabetes control?

VIRGINIA: Yes. Lois is a patient who has the enviable life of spending half the year in Albuquerque and the other half on a lake in Michigan. (You get to guess which half where.) She has done an incredible job of managing her diabetes with exercise and diet. My partner LaVerne first started working with Lois while she was on insulin. With daily exercise Lois was able to lose 50 pounds and now has perfect blood sugars with no medications. She enjoys hosting students in her home who come to Michigan for music camp, including my daughter Melanie, who says, "Lois is rad."

So it's agreed, exercise makes all our diabetes goals easier to achieve, but how can you make exercise itself easier? That's my problem. Although I love Covert Bailey, he hasn't been able to seduce me yet.

JUNE AND BARBARA: You just start exercising. To begin, take whatever baby steps you have to—even if you exercise only four or five minutes a day. *Thinking* about exercising is what's hard. If you start doing something—almost anything—you're on your way. You've probably heard the saying, "appetite comes with eating." Well, motivation to exercise comes with exercising.

Of course, there are some strategies and tricks you can use to get you going and keep you at it. The first strategy is to block out a time slot. Any time is great, though some experts especially recommend walking after meals. Back when we were working long hours in the SugarFree Center, the only way we could get in our exercise on weekdays was to do it right after breakfast. June did one half hour on a Schwinn Aerodyne (which provides both arm and leg exercise) and Barbara did a half hour of aerobics on a trampoline. On the weekends we would bike or walk. Now that we aren't tied down to an 8:00 A.M. to 5:00 or 6:00 P.M. schedule (we can just work all the time, weekends and holidays included), we try to walk three or four miles after breakfast three or four days a week and to go to the gym for upper body strengthening at least two days a week. We try to go to the gym at 1:00 P.M. because at other times the machines are crowded and we're too impatient to stand around and wait. Early Sunday mornings is also an ideal time since most of the workout-crazed yuppies are sleeping in after their big Saturday nights.

What we're trying to emphasize here is that you should work out your time schedule to fit your own life and sports activities. Everyone can do it! If you have to cut down on your time reading the newspaper or chatting on the telephone or playing bridge or watching TV, that's what you do.

Actually, cutting down on TV-watching is one of the best things you can do for yourself. A recent *New York Times* article told of a study by psychologist Robert Klesges of Memphis State University. He discovered that when children watch television, "they lapse into a deeply relaxed, almost semi conscious state . . . between resting and sleeping." This lowers their metabolic rate so that these children burn fewer calories watching TV than they would if they sat still doing nothing and almost as few as if they were sleeping.

Dr. Klesges believes that this TV-induced drop in metabolic rate could be a major contributor to obesity. In other words, it's the opposite of Covert Bailey's exercise-induced revving up of the metabolism. So cut down on TV-watching. It will prevent softening of the body as well as softening of the brain.

But whatever other activity you have to give up, just don't chicken out with that tired old excuse, "I have no time for exercise."

VIRGINIA: You're getting awfully serious about this. OK, I'll find a way to make the time. But I confess that I'm still reluctant. You said it was easy to get yourself in motion.

JUNE AND BARBARA: Maybe you're reluctant because you have no specific goals. Nothing is accomplished if you don't figure out beforehand exactly what it is that you want to accomplish. So here's our pitch on goals.

Set short-term goals by the week.
Your goal must be specific, concrete, and realistically ambitious. (You can read about the art of setting goals in our book *Psyching Out Diabetes,* written with Dr. Richard Rubin.) A main point to remember is that the goal must be one you really want to reach. It won't work to let your spouse or even your doctor set your goal. If you set it, you're much more likely to accomplish it. It's OK to let your friends and family know your goal, as they may be able to help you stick with it.

Don't set your goals too high.
This is another of the basic rules of goal setting. If you're thinking of jogging, for instance, you begin with half-mile runs, and then eventually you might want to work up to something as grandiose as 5 miles per week and in a few years 20 miles per week. All the new books on exercise emphasize that you should start out slow; the more out-of-shape you are, the slower you should start out. In fact, we've heard that to get in shape, it takes a month for every year you've been out of shape. For some of us that adds up to quite a chunk of time.

Have a goal of do-it-every-day.
For people with diabetes, it is preferable to have the goal of exercising every day rather than the usual three or four times a week idea that has been so prominent in health advice. This is because it's easier to balance your medication and adjust your diet with daily activity. (There are exceptions, which we will explain.) One excellent walking program, *Walking Off Weight,* by Robert Sweetgall, Roba Whiteley, and Robert Neeves, advocates an eight-days-a-week goal, and that means walking not only every day but sometimes twice in one day so that if you miss a day occasionally, you'll still have done seven workouts a week.

Covert Bailey, who 16 years ago was preaching his 12 minutes of aerobic exercise three times a week as a total program, has switched to new advice: "exercise longer, not harder." He has learned that his original method of having people use the formula 220 minus their age to get their maximum heart rate to set their exercise target zone is not effective for about 40 percent of the population and was causing a lot of people to overdo or underdo.

(Approximately 15 percent of people have a slower heartbeat than the average and 15 percent have a faster heartbeat.) Now he emphasizes that "exercising at low levels is far, far more beneficial than we originally thought." One of his new rules is to "exercise as much as possible." And he's recommending that even beginners exercise six times a week for 12 minutes.

We might sum up by saying that your goal should be to try to get some exercise every day, even if it's only a few minutes and even if it's done in more than one short session. (See how reasonable we are?) As cardiologist James Rippe, director of the University of Massachusetts Medical School Exercise Physiology Lab, says, "You don't have to turn your life upside down to do things that have a profound impact on how happy, productive, and healthy you are." He recommends a simple two-step plan to feel better and reduce risk of heart disease: (1) Eat cereal with skim milk for breakfast, then (2) go out for a 15-minute walk. This simple plan works just as well for people with diabetes.

VIRGINIA: What a relief to know that I don't have to aim for exercise workouts that leave me sweating and panting and exhausted. I'm getting a little more enthusiastic. Do you have any more motivators in your gym bag?

JUNE AND BARBARA: We always have more! To impress yourself with your spectacular progress in fulfilling your goals, keep records, or as the sportspeople call it, a log book. These records can be as simple as jotting down the day of the week, the time of day, the kind of exercise, and the length of time you exercised. You can use an ordinary monthly calendar with large squares for each day. Or if you keep blood sugar and medications records in one of the log books provided by meter companies, add your exercise record to this.

At the end of each week, total your time and see if you achieved your goal or how close you came to it. Maybe you even surpassed your goal and you can crow about it.

VIRGINIA: That's easy enough. When do we get to the hard part?

JUNE AND BARBARA: There really isn't any hard part—except maybe in certain people's minds. What we're coming to now is the *easiest* part—the reward or celebration for achieving your goal. We ourselves have gotten this down to a science. We have a reward not every week, month, or year but *every day.* This is the way it works. It's two miles from our house to the Coffee Roaster on famous Ventura Boulevard in the San Fernando Valley (just over the hill from the more famous Hollywood Boulevard). The Coffee Roaster is the neighborhood vendor of freshly roasted choice gourmet coffee beans, featuring outstanding cups of coffee, cappuccinos, and espressos and featuring owner Dick Healy's own fresh, home-baked fruit muffins (low in sugar and moderate in size). June takes her blood sugar—it's usually low after the two-mile walk—and then she's eligible for the reward: coffee and a blueberry, cherry walnut, or peach muffin, whatever is in season. The muffin—or sometimes half of one—is just enough fuel to sustain a Type II-D diabetic like her for the two-mile return trip. (Type II-R's might have coffee or tea, maybe with artificial sweetener, or a cappuccino made with nonfat milk.) On gym days we have an alternate but equally delightful reward.

So all you do is find a spot that's far enough away, a spot with something good to drink and/or eat, and take off. If you don't live in an area as coffeehouse filled as ours or don't like coffee or tea, you can carry your reward in your backpack and sit and enjoy it at the midpoint of your walk. This is just one idea. There are many nonfood rewards, even such schemes as putting 10 cents in a piggy bank for every mile or minute you walk. This is also a good way of keeping track of how long you exercise each day. The money saved this way is, of course, a discretionary fund to spend in any wild and crazy and impractical way you choose.

There are probably some saintly people out there who don't even crave such material rewards. Their reward is the inner satisfaction of achieving their goal and feeling healthier and more energetic, looking better and enjoying life more.

VIRGINIA: You're right about the importance of goals. Almost all successful people work with goals and rewards. I'm sitting here wondering, though, about the next problem that has popped into my mind. What kind of exercise are Type II's going to do? As we teach at The Presbyterian Diabetes Center, the activity should be aerobic, which is defined as continuous, rhythmic exercise done at a level that feels somewhat difficult. This means walking, jogging, running, bicycling, rowing, swimming, jumping rope, aerobic dancing, roller skating, treadmill walking. . . .

JUNE AND BARBARA: Aerobic is the word, all right. And you've given us the main choices, except maybe cross-country skiing, which is the most intensive workout of all. Your selection of sport is controlled to some extent by where you're going to be exercising: at home, in your neighborhood, or in a fitness center or gym. The aerobic possibilities in each of these locations differ.

In your home
If you can't leave the house because of weather, small children, hazardous neighborhood, or physical problems, then your exercise will depend largely on in-house equipment. You buy what you like and what you can afford. We've mentioned trampolines and jumping ropes, both inexpensive but quite intensive. More pricey (in order of least expensive) to most expensive are rowing machines, cross-country skiing machines, exercycles, treadmills, and stair-climbing machines. A good treadmill can set you back a pretty penny, say, $1,200 to $3,000. The popular stair climbers or step machines cost up to $5,000. (June's orthopedist warns against the stair-climbers because they're too hard on the knees.)

In judging equipment you have to be certain that you aren't going for something that will stress your back problem or your bad elbow or whatever other physical injuries or debilities you may have. There's a lot to think about, so be wary of fast-talking salespeople who are themselves athletic types and don't understand that all of us are not as young and or in as prime physical condition as they are.

Last there is the gentlest, least-damaging exercise of them all, swimming. If your house already has a pool, fine. If not, prepare for an investment of something like the equivalent of a first-class trip around the world or the purchase of a new Cadillac. A new swimming pool exercise we've just heard about is "water walking"—walking in the pool. The resistance of the water multiplies the effectiveness of your exercise.

In your neighborhood
Neighborhood exercise choices including walking, jogging, biking, and, for those who live in snowy country, cross-country skiing in winter. You can also look for a public swimming pool in your neighborhood. Some condo complexes allow nonresidents to use their pools for a membership fee.

In a fitness center or gym
Almost all modern fitness centers have aerobic exercise available as well as weights and Nautilus-style machines for muscle-strengthening exercises. At the LA Fitness gym where we go, the trainers want you to warm up for at least 20 minutes on the aerobic equipment before you begin your strength training workout. Not a bad idea, because a little of each is always better than a lot of either.

The advantage of the gym is that you can go in any weather and do a variety of exercises; the disadvantage is that at certain hours, especially early mornings and evenings, they are overcrowded and you have to waste time waiting to use the equipment. Ask the attendants which hours are the least popular and see if you can't work your schedule around those times.

The other leading disadvantage is the cost. The initial fee can be as low as free if the company is running an advertised special or it could be up to $150. There is a monthly charge of maybe $25 to $50, depending on your neighborhood (high-rent areas charge the most); often family members can sign on together for lower rates. Be sure to investigate the company, as lots of scammy stuff goes on with some of these chains. The gym may go out of business after you've paid a big up-front fee, or it may sell out to another organization that won't honor your initial contract.

Now comes the big decision. You've picked your main workout location, so which particular sports are you going to go for? Here are some guidelines:

- Choose the exercises that most appeal to you.
- Choose the exercises you can do most often.
- Choose more than one exercise, especially if you're older, so that you can alternate them and give different muscles time to recoup between sessions.

- Choose aerobic exercise, but add some form of muscle-strengthening exercise. Sixty-five percent of the body's muscles are above the hips and most aerobic exercises do little to strengthen them.
- Choose some load-bearing exercise. For example, if swimming is your main thing, also do some activity in which you're on your feet. This is especially important for women because it helps avoid osteoporosis.

VIRGINIA: That sounds like an ideal plan, but you know many of us will be lucky to get into *one* form of exercise. And some of us Type II-R's need a little extra nudge to put us on the right track. Couldn't you give us at least a hint about which exercise would be the easiest and least likely to defeat us in the beginning?

JUNE AND BARBARA: That's exactly what we were hoping you would ask. The answer is clear and unequivocal: walking. To quote the albeit somewhat prejudiced author of a book on walking, Casey Meyers, "Walking is the most injury-free, sustainable, effective, complete exercise" there is. He also claims it uses more energy and burns more calories than running. Furthermore, Meyers proves via research that humans are biomechanically engineered to be walkers, not runners. As he puts it, "If God had meant humans to run, He would have given us the locomotion system of a horse."

Walking's our all-time favorite. Though we do other sports off and on, it's the activity we've most successfully woven into the fabric of our lives. It's a low-impact, lifetime exercise. You can do it fast (4 miles an hour) or slow (2 miles an hour). It's quick, convenient, and inexpensive. You can do it alone, with one other person, or in a group. Group and individual mallwalking programs are now available for people of all ages in some shopping centers. In our neighborhood there are two walking tracks in two parks and we see people out doing their fitness walks at all hours of the day (except when it's 100 degrees).

Walking is also a perfect vacation sight-seeing activity. This year we spent 10 days walking all over Florence and two weeks walking streets and roads and trails in the area around Montreux, Switzerland.

Walking is the least expensive exercise, especially compared to such equipment-intensive sports as golfing, aerobics classes, tennis, and skiing. But there are a couple of things you do have to invest a bit of money in: shoes and socks. For a person with diabetes, choosing these isn't exactly a simple matter. We say this because of the amount of attention that must be paid to the legendary "diabetic foot." You find long lists of do's and don'ts about foot care in all diabetes manuals. We were surprised when one of our own books was indexed with a heading "diabetic foot," because no other part of the diabetic body was so listed. There was no entry for the diabetic thumb or ear. It's as if when you have diabetes, your Achilles heel is a whole Achilles foot. Virginia, here is where you come in. Can you explain why diabetic feet are different from ordinary feet?

VIRGINIA: Actually, diabetic feet start out like normal feet, but suffer the effects of the disease as time goes by. When glucose levels stay above normal—over 180–200—year after year, two different problems add up to serious changes in the feet.

The first problem is the decrease in circulation that can occur because of diabetes. Excess glucose and excess insulin work together to plug up your blood vessels. Poor circulation in your feet and legs means that they can't respond to the stress of a little sore by combating germs and infections. Your feet cannot heal the way normal feet do.

The second problem is the damage to nerves that high blood sugar can cause. When the nerves serving your feet and legs are damaged, they act like a faulty electrical circuit. First, you get static—tingling, strange shooting pains—and eventually numbness. This may seem like a relief after the tingling and pain, but it's very dangerous, because you don't know when you're getting the kind of excessive pressure that causes blisters, or you may be unaware that you've stepped on a tack. Eventually you could end up with structural deformities of the foot, because it is the nerves that keep the muscles stimulated to hold your feet in shape.

This is why diabetic feet need special tender loving care.

JUNE AND BARBARA: And that's the reason we're going to go into detail about purchasing shoes and socks. Not that everyone—with diabetes or not—who is an avid walker or jogger shouldn't be concerned about choosing the right foot attire. You can't enjoy walking unless your feet feel good both during and after. And it's not easy to make your selection these days since there is a proliferation of walking and running shoes and all the major brands have some new technology to hype: Nike has Air and Anatomical Arch Supports; Avia has Clear Cantilever outsole and ArchRocker; Reebok has its Dynamic Cushioning System; Brooks has its Propulsion Plate System and HydroFlow cushioning. Something new comes along every day, and the buyer has to be wary.

Not only is there controversy about all this fancy technology, but there is little agreement about whether you should buy shoes designed specifically for walking or shoes specifically designed for running. We personally go for running shoes since the tread is usually more pronounced and therefore cushions and grips better. Robert Sweetgall says you should make sure that the shoes do not have flat bottoms. They should have a rocker profile; you ought to be able to see daylight under the toes and heels.

VIRGINIA: I especially like my Asics Gels for their cushioned support.

JUNE AND BARBARA: Then you agree with the experts who say that comfort is all. We advise people to go to a sports shoe shop, where the salespeople are often fanatical walkers or runners themselves and may know more and care more than the department store shoe salesperson. You should insist on a choice of several different brands and you should try each on and walk around a bit—even go outdoors and try them on the sidewalk— until you can decide on the most comfortable. Above all, do not settle for anything but your own size (some salespeople will try to peddle what they have in stock, even if it's a half-size too short or long or narrower or wider than you require). You should have a thumb width between the end of your toe and the end of the shoe. And a word to women: don't worry about looks. These are not things of beauty, but sports shoes are in style now all over America, so just change your thinking about what is attractive on your feet.

What are these ideally comfortable and well-fitting walking or running shoes going to cost? More than you'll want to pay for a pair for yourself (especially if you're a woman), but about what you would be willing to pay for a pair for your kid. Sixty or seventy dollars is not outrageous. The bad news is that when you get into walking 20 or so miles a week, you'll need to toss out the old and bring in the new every six months. As one sports shoe expert told us, you wouldn't want to drive around on worn-out tires with no tread. It's just as bad to walk around on worn-out shoes with no tread. One little money-saving tip is that sometimes you can pick up the previous model of a newly redesigned shoe at lesser cost than the latest version. New models come on the market so frequently that the previous one is usually just as good structurally as the latest edition.

Now for the socks. Seven or eight dollars a pair will buy you socks that will help prevent blisters and/or give you extra padding on the ball of the foot where you might have pain if your fat pad has grown thin over the years or if you tend to build up calluses. As verified by a study in *Diabetes Medicine,* this extra padding may also prevent diabetic foot problems by reducing the pressure on the vulnerable parts of the foot.

The brands we use are Double Lay'R socks (for blister prevention; very soft and nice) and Thor-Lo athletic socks, which have extra knitting at heel and ball areas. Thor-Lo makes many kinds of athletic socks (tennis, golf, aerobics, etc.), so make sure you get walking socks. Both these brands are available in sports shoe shops and also mail order from the manufacturer (Double Lay'R is 1-800-392-8500; Thor-Lo is 1-800-457-2256).

VIRGINIA: I'd like to add that when buying your shoes you should wear your padded socks. And I like stores whose salespeople know how to fit you the old-fashioned way. Remember when you were a kid, the salesperson would feel the shoe and tell you whether or not it fit? If you have "at risk" feet, you have diminished sensation and you can't trust your feet to tell you how well the shoe fits. It's not worth saving a few dollars at a discount self-serve shoe store and losing a foot!

Now how about telling us how walking becomes an aerobic exercise in the sense that it strengthens the heart and helps control blood pressure?

JUNE AND BARBARA: You have to walk fast enough to increase your heart rate (number of beats per minute) to at least 65 percent of its maximum rate. That means you have to walk a mile in about 17 minutes. The standard way of figuring your maximum heart rate is easy: subtract your age from the number 220. For instance, if you're 55, the formula is 220 − 55 = 165 beats per minute. (You definitely don't want to reach that rate during exercise.) Then take 65 percent of 165 and you get 107 beats per minute. That's your "target rate," but most of you will have to consider your age and physical condition and approach that target slowly. Also, remember Covert Bailey's caution that this formula may not apply to you individually, so you might want to check with your doctor.

To monitor your pulse, check it before, during, and after exercise. Using your fingertips, find your pulse at your wrist (inside) or at the carotid artery underneath your jawbone at the left side of your neck. Count for 10 seconds and multiply by 6 to get your heartbeats per minute. (Our guru Covert Bailey prefers that you count for 6 seconds and multiply by 10; this does make multiplying easier, but it's harder to count for exactly 6 seconds because it's such a short time.)

The goal is to keep your heart rate at its target of 60 percent for about 20 to 30 minutes at a time. Only a sustained, uninterrupted effort for this amount of time can condition your heart. This kind of continuous, rhythmical exercise that uses the muscles of the lower body is what's called aerobic exercise. Walking, of course, is only one of many such exercises. You can choose from bicycling, swimming, jogging, aerobic dancing, roller skating, jumping rope, and others.

VIRGINIA: I get the picture, and I know you start out slowly, with your doctor's approval, if you haven't been doing much of anything in the exercise line. As far as diabetes is concerned, I have to recommend also that you not only monitor your heart rate, but you also monitor your blood sugar if you take pills or

insulin, especially insulin. Your blood sugar should be at least 150
before you start your exercise session. If it's less, eat a snack
before starting. If it's over 250, there's another factor to consider.
There may not be adequate insulin on board to handle the
increased demand for fuel that will occur with exercise, and your
blood sugar will go up even higher.

In helping patients set up an exercise program I always explain
that they should do their exercise for at least 20 to 30 minutes at a
time at least three or four times a week. It should be done at a
level that feels somewhat difficult, but not so strenuously that you
feel out of breath. And above all, don't exceed your target heart
range.

BARBARA AND JUNE: We hate to remind you that aerobic
activity is not the end of the exercise program anymore. All the
experts claim now, and we certainly go along with them, that aerobics alone are not enough. You must also do some strength training.

VIRGINIA: You mean pumping iron? Who wants big biceps and
show-off muscles? I certainly don't want to look like Popeye and
not many of my patients do either.

JUNE AND BARBARA: Don't get us wrong. We don't either.
What is being advocated for health benefits has nothing to do with
professional body building. Strength training is done by lifting
hand-held weights or using weight machines like Nautilus. It's
been shown that this kind of training retards the aging process—
and you can't knock that. It can make a 90-year-old as strong as a
50-year-old. But the biggest news is that besides reducing the risk
of getting diabetes, it improves insulin sensitivity, and that should
make it especially popular with all Type II-R's.

VIRGINIA: Come to think of it, it has another great advantage: it
improves the body's proportion of muscle to fat, and this really
counts from a health standpoint. If your body has a high percentage of fat, it does not require as many calories to preserve that fat.
The result is that when you eat extra calories, the body stores

them with all that other fat. This is not good news unless you're preparing for a famine. So by converting fat to muscle you can change your metabolism so that you burn more calories. This, of course, helps solve weight problems.

JUNE AND BARBARA: That's why some health professionals think recommended weight should be determined by measuring the proportion of fat and lean tissue. They don't consider the old height-weight tables good guides. Wouldn't it be good news to find out that your weightiness was mostly due to muscle and therefore not a health risk at all? Muscle weighs more than fat, so you can see why you could be heavy with muscle and have a high total weight, but not be unhealthy.

The recommended proportion of body fat is different for men and women. Men should be between 6 and 23 percent fat and women between 9 and 30 percent. Men who are 25 percent fat and women who are 35 percent fat are classified as obese. Covert Bailey wants men to be not over 15 percent fat and women not over 22 percent.

The most accurate body-composition test is naturally the most awkward and expensive. For it, you must be weighed under water using a hydrosensitomer. Since fat floats and muscle sinks, the heavier you are under water, the better. (It's the opposite of the situation on land!) An easier test is to find a doctor or gym that has a Futrex-5000 Bodyfat Analyzer. This measures the percentage of fat with a near-infrared light beam that is sent into your most prominent biceps. The instrument prints out a detailed analysis of your fitness state and a program for improvement. The simplest method is a caliper test in your doctor's office or a fitness center. For a rough idea, you can pinch up your flesh just below the ribs at your waistline. You should find a thickness of between one-half and one inch. If there's more flesh than that, you're too fat, even if the scales don't tell you so.

VIRGINIA: Okay, let's get back to muscle building. You've made your point. How do you get going on it and how do you learn how to do it?

JUNE AND BARBARA: It's not as hard as you may think. You don't even have to grunt. In fact, you shouldn't exert yourself that much. And you only have to do it about twice a week. We usually alternate it with our walking exercise, as you don't want to do strength training two days in a row. Your muscles like to rest.

VIRGINIA: Well, I don't have a gym in the mountains where I live. Does that mean I can't do muscle strengthening?

JUNE AND BARBARA: No, it just means you do it at home using free weights. The main problem with that is that, unless the Presbyterian Diabetes Center has an exercise therapist on staff, you'll have to find one to visit or you'll have to buy one of the better books on weightlifting. Two of these are *Designing Resistance Training Programs* by S. J. Fleck and W. J. Kraemer (Champaigne, IL: Human Kinetics Books, 1987); and *Lift Your Way to Youthful Fitness* by Jerry Todd and Jan Todd (Boston: Little, Brown, 1985).

We're lucky because there are plenty of gyms in Southern California and when we're free to go at uncrowded hours we can get an excellent workout in a short time. There's something motivating about a gym. A "Personal Health" column in the *Los Angeles Times* about sticking with exercise revealed that women need social support to adopt and maintain an exercise program, while men are motivated by a favorable environment. In a gym you do fraternize with the other exercisers and the environment is more than favorable, because you can't do anything but exercise while you're there. And we find it fun to learn to use the fancy new fitness machines. Our gym has Nautilus and Cybex equipment. The latter are easy to set, smooth to use, and make you feel like a real pro.

When you join a gym you usually get at least one complimentary lesson with a trainer who designs a program just for you. But you have to watch out when signing on, as gyms are now a big business and a very competitive one and some firms have indulged in fraudulent activities, like signing up hundreds of people and then going out of business or charging excessive start-up fees with the hope that you'll sign on and then drop out within a few months. All have aggressive sales staffs to push you into signing a contract. So beware; you've been warned.

VIRGINIA: Can you give us a brief glimpse of what you actually do during a workout? Some people have never been inside a gym. And are there any cautions for persons with diabetes?

JUNE AND BARBARA: You're supposed to work at least 8 or 10 different muscle groups and do one set of each exercise. A set is 10 to 12 repetitions. For instance, we do abdominal, back extension, arm curl, rowing, chest press, lateral pulldown, lateral rise, leg extension, leg curl, and hip adduction. (Those terms are probably mysterious to you, because you have to see the machines to know what they mean.) The load you set the machine for (in 5- or 10-pound increments) has to be light enough so that you can lift it at least 8 times before your muscles fatigue. If you can lift it more than 15 times, it's too light. You work up to about 30 repetitions and then you go on to the next heavier weight.

VIRGINIA: How do you keep from injuring yourself? I've known people who strained muscles in gyms.

JUNE AND BARBARA: Experts William Evans, chief of the Human Physiology Laboratory at the Human Nutrition Research Center on Aging at Tufts University, and Michael Preuss, fitness director at Cooper Aerobics Center in Dallas, give these cautions:

- Lift slowly, avoiding jerky or "explosive" movements. Lifting a weight should take two or three seconds; lowering it should take about the same amount of time.
- Ask a trainer in the health club to demonstrate proper breathing technique.
- Ask your doctor's advice or get an examination before beginning, especially if you're older or have diabetes or high blood pressure.
- Don't go overboard. An every-other-day program works best.

We would alter that last caution to once or twice a week. And if you have proliferative diabetic retinopathy (a disease of the retina), weight training is a great risk. In fact, get permission from your ophthalmologist if you have even moderate retinopathy. Also talk to your doctor if you have chronic hypertension.

VIRGINIA: I think I need to go rest now. Do you have any final words about exercise?

JUNE AND BARBARA: We have a final story about weightlifting that we know you'd like to hear.

We read an article in the May 1992 *Diabetes Forecast* that profiled Ron Gillembardo of Las Vegas. Ron was diagnosed with Type II diabetes in 1982 when he was 38 years old. His blood sugar was 500 and he tipped the scales at 360 pounds. He started working out with weights and he just happened to excel at it. In less than two years he lost nearly 100 pounds and he got off insulin and onto pills. He kept working out with weights two hours a day, five days a week.

In 1989 Ron began powerlifting in competitions. He won almost every competition he entered and became the world record holder in the 710-pound lift. Last year at the age of 43 he qualified for the 1992 Olympic Games in Barcelona. He is the oldest weightlifter ever to compete in the Olympics.

Now doesn't that make you want to get out there and see what kind of prizes you can win with exercise? The best prize, of course, will be your wonderful diabetes control and your new self-esteem.

CHAPTER 4

FOOD, DIET, NUTRITION: THE "ONLY MORE SO" DISEASE

People with diabetes are not that different from the rest of the population. When you come right down to it, for optimum health, a person with Type II diabetes needs to do what anyone else should do—only more so. Everybody needs to be on an exercise program; so does the person with diabetes—only more so. All inhabitants of the modern world need to learn how to handle personal and work and societal stresses; so does the person with diabetes—only more so.

In no area does the "only more so" factor apply more strongly than in diet. From reports issued by the Surgeon General, the National Institutes of Health, the American Heart Association, and the American Cancer Society, we know that everyone needs to drastically cut back on fat and sweets and overrefined carbohydrates and add more fiber to their diets. So does the person with diabetes—only more so, very much more so.

What we all need to do is return to the diet and lifestyle that our genes were designed for and our bodies were built for. *The Paleolithic Prescription,* a book by Atlanta radiologist Boyd Eaton, M.D., and Emory University anthropology professors Melvin Konner and Marjorie Shostak, tells us that our genes cry out for the Stone Age cuisine that our primitive ancestors served up in their cavernous family rooms 40,000 years ago.

They maintain that most of the illnesses of civilization—
heart disease, osteoporosis, cancer, and good old diabetes—are caused by our eating a diet our bodies
weren't designed for.

The primitive diet consisted of mainly wild vegetables, fruits, and game. The "wild" part is significant.
The wild fruits and vegetables were much richer in vitamins, minerals, and fiber than the modern domesticat-
ed varieties, and since they were usually chomped
down raw, the food values weren't diminished in cook-
ing. Wild game is far leaner than the farm-bred, corn-
fed meat we find in the market. This was vividly demon-
strated to us when a friend invited us to partake of wild
goose that her Idaho hunter son had sent her.
Fatophobe June cringed at the thought, because all of
her past roast goose experiences had been with creatures that oozed enough grease to provide oil for all the
lamps of China. But this turned out to be the leanest
serving of protein she'd ever consumed. The small
amount of fat that wild game does contain is proportion-
ately lower in the harmful saturated variety than farm-
raised meat.

Since we obviously can't go back to gathering our
own wild vegetables and chasing down game, we need
a modern "Paleolithic Prescription" that we can fill for
ourselves. Because there is far less fiber in our cultivat-
ed fruits and vegetables, we need to get more of our
fiber from cereals and breads. (Our primitive ancestors,
who weren't cultivators, didn't have such foods.)
Particularly important are the soluble fibers from oat
and corn products since they reduce serum cholesterol.
A fiber supplement is also a great diet insurance policy,
especially for people who eat out frequently or use a lot
of processed foods.

The animal protein should be of the low-fat variety—
fish is particularly good. Low- or nonfat dairy products
are an inexpensive source of protein plus calcium. We
need more calcium because our vegetables of today
contain much less than their wild forebears. For this

reason the Paleolithic Prescribers advise a calcium supplement to help prevent osteoporosis, high blood pressure, and colon cancer. They particularly recommend calcium carbonate because that's the most easily absorbed form of the mineral.

So use the Primitive Diet as your basic guideline and combine with it the variations Virginia will explain as most suitable to your particular kind of Type II diabetes, and you will find that before long you'll look and feel as healthy, vital, and vibrant as your nondiabetic contemporaries—only more so!

—June and Barbara

What You'll Find in This Chapter

The "Fast Fast"
Low-Fat Lifestyle
Restaurant Dining
Binge Eating
Carbohydrates
Glycemic Index
Fiber
Snacking

JUNE AND BARBARA: When people are diagnosed with Type II diabetes, they're usually told that with a little bit of luck they can probably control their blood sugar level simply by changing their diet and adding regular exercise. This is a comforting thought, compared with taking blood-sugar–lowering pills or injections of insulin, but is it true?

VIRGINIA: Yes, Type II-R diabetes can be managed with diet and weight loss in many cases. Statistics tell us that among people with Type II-R diabetes, one-third control their diabetes with diet, one-third with pills, and one-third with insulin. Does this mean that two-thirds of all Type II-R's are bad people who don't follow a proper diet? No, these statistics probably reflect the evolution of the disease.

Initially, the disease is manifested primarily in insulin resistance and is amenable to treatment with diet and exercise. As the insulin deficiency becomes more severe, the need for oral agents and insulin increases. Eventually, when the insulin deficiency and excessive liver glucose production outstrip the pills' ability to control blood sugars, insulin becomes essential.

For many people the Presbyterian Diabetes Center suggests what we call the Fast Fast to help people get their blood sugars into control quickly, or to get off medications if they're already using them.

The Fast Fast is not really a fast. It's a fast from carbohydrates only. (All foods are composed of various combinations of carbohydrate, protein, and fat; carbohydrates are sugars and starches and they usually account for about 50 percent of what we eat.) On the Fast Fast you can eat as much salad with low-fat dressing as you want. You eat at least one small meat serving a day, baked, broiled or boiled, and all the sugar-free gelatin you can stand, any color. You can also have all the sugar-free sodas, coffee, and tea you want, but on top of that you should be sure to drink at least eight large glasses of water a day.

JUNE AND BARBARA: How do most people feel while on the Fast Fast?

VIRGINIA: They usually don't feel bad at all. What happens is that they get a headache the first day and then they're not even hungry after that.

We always have people on the Fast Fast test their blood sugar at least twice a day, because blood sugars can drop precipitously. People on insulin or pills will need a health professional to coach them so they know how to decrease their medication in anticipation of the lowering blood sugars. Otherwise they might get too low and run out and attack a donut shop or something. To get off the pills or insulin and achieve the goal glucose level takes three to five days. Then you start adding carbohydrates . . . slowly. First add low-carbohydrate green vegetables such as green beans, broccoli, spinach, and the like. Even though they're green, peas are almost pure starch, so don't add them yet. Avocados are high in fat, so don't add them. Next try adding toast for breakfast, then maybe a potato at dinner. In other words, gradually add one carbohydrate at a time to see the effect on your blood sugar.

Let me tell you about Mary Jane, a nurse who works nights and has had Type II diabetes for 8 or 10 years. She was one of the students in a nursing course I was teaching for the University of Phoenix in Albuquerque. She introduced herself, rather proudly, as a "noncompliant" diabetic. (At the time, she was unaware of what I did for a living.) She was a typical picture of a person with diabetes who had been blamed for her disease for so long that she pinned the"noncompliant" label on herself before anyone else had a chance to. She was 75 pounds overweight, taking large amounts of insulin, but still her blood glucose levels usually ran from 200 to 400. She felt bad all the time and she felt helpless to stop her cycle of overeating and poor control. Worst of all, she believed her problems were all her own fault.

After we had known each other for a few weeks, Mary Jane came up to me after class and described how she would wake up with low blood sugar every afternoon and eat the house down for the rest of the evening. Then she'd go to work at 10:30 P.M. and feel awful. (Her insulin regimen was the same as if she had been on a day schedule.) I asked her to let me know when she was ready to get off insulin and I would help her.

She waited a few weeks before she brought up the subject. I told her how to do the Fast Fast, lowering her insulin as her blood glucose levels came down. (Since she was a nurse, she could be trusted to handle this on her own.) She called me on the weekend to complain that she felt awful. She wasn't used to having blood glucose levels in the normal range; of course, she felt entirely different from when she was 200 to 300 all the time. But even though she felt bad, boy, was she excited and happy because *she was off insulin!*

She had an appointment with her doctor for that next week. I told her to ask him for a prescription for an oral hypoglycemic agent so that if her blood glucose levels started going up a little as she gradually added back carbohydrate food, she would have a safety net. We also spent a great deal of time talking about how to eat light, low-fat meals and about starting to exercise.

Her doctor was shocked that she was off insulin and that her fasting blood glucose was down to 185. (She would get lower than that throughout the day, but that pesky liver would pop it up during the night, and that's why she needed the pills.) The doctor suggested she go back on insulin, and Mary Jane rightly replied, "Remember what my blood glucose level was when I was on insulin?" On top of that, she was now 12 pounds lighter. By taking Diabeta pills (she calls them Diabetter) and getting back on carbohydrates, she is keeping her blood glucose levels between 100 and 200 and has lost a total of 35 pounds. She's exercising at least three hours a week and is feeling better than she has in years.

JUNE AND BARBARA: The Fast Fast sounds like a miracle cure, but Mary Jane had had diabetes for 8 or 10 years. Does the Fast Fast work equally well for newly diagnosed diabetics?

VIRGINIA: Yes, I have another success story for you that proves it. I met Nick in the hospital. His doctor had hospitalized him as a newly diagnosed diabetic, though most endocrinologists, instead of putting patients in the hospital, let us at the Presbyterian Diabetes Center do their initial training and glucose control as outpatients. Nick, a good-looking though chubby Hispanic guy about 35 years old, is a computer operator who leads a pretty sedentary life. He had gone to the doctor with symptoms of excess urination, excess thirst, and generally feeling awful. He suspected diabetes, because most of the people in his family over the age of 60 had the disease. He had not lost large amounts of weight during this period of illness. In fact, he was about 50 pounds overweight.

The doctor had him on 70/30 insulin (NPH and Regular premixed in a vial) and wanted him to get a blood glucose testing meter. I was to teach him how to use the meter. His blood sugars were still moderately high, in the 200s. I told him that it would be useful to him to be on insulin, because otherwise his health insurance would not pay for the meter. But I promised him that we could get him off insulin pronto, whenever he was ready. He looked at me as if I were crazy. I think the doctor must have told him I *was* crazy, because we didn't see him again at the Center for a few months.

He finally decided to come to our eight-week course. He was still on insulin, but his dose was lower. He had lost about 10 pounds, because his wife was following the diet guidelines given to them in the hospital. When he showed up in class, he asked me about getting off insulin. I said, "Sure, Nick, whenever you're ready." I knew it wouldn't be difficult, because he was on so little insulin—about 16 units in the morning and 10 units at night. For a guy weighing over 200 pounds, if he really needed insulin, it would have taken a lot more than that. Besides, when you're young and brand-new to diabetes, the Fast Fast works especially well.

He started on the Fast and in a few days was normoglycemic (another word for euglycemic) and off of insulin.

JUNE AND BARBARA: We're happy to hear you talk about people getting off insulin. There's a terrible rumor going around that once you start taking insulin you have to take it forever. One Type II woman, who had always been controlled with diet and exercise, wrote and told us of what was a terrifying experience for her. She had been hospitalized for surgery and the stress caused her blood sugars to go up. When her doctors told her they were going to give her some insulin to bring it down, she fainted dead away. That was because she thought she was going to be on insulin for the rest of her life. After her recovery, her blood sugar went back down and she could again control her diabetes without insulin. "But," she complained, "why did I have to go through that when it wasn't necessary? Why didn't someone explain to me that this was just a temporary thing?" Why indeed? Let's hear it for letting the patient know what's going on! But how about Nick? Is he still off insulin?

VIRGINIA: Yes, he's continued to keep his blood glucose in control with diet. He has a nice blood glucose meter to keep track of it, thanks to his health insurance. If Nick can keep losing weight, he'll probably be able to control his diabetes for many years with diet and exercise. This is not to say that the disease was solely caused by his diet, his obesity, or his sedentary lifestyle. Those factors were certainly not in his favor, but we know lots of guys just like Nick—overweight, sedentary lifestyle—who don't have diabetes. Remember Type II-R diabetes is a genetic disease, not a character flaw!

JUNE AND BARBARA: Some doctors advocate that people with diabetes control their blood sugar by staying permanently on a high-protein diet. The rationale is that by eating mostly protein (fish, chicken, meat, cheese) and eating the right number of calories, the person can avoid the surges of glucose that carbohydrates cause. The high-protein diet is the basis of Dr. Richard K. Bernstein's method of normalizing blood sugar permanently for Type II diabetics. It's spelled out in his book, *Diabetes Type II*. We take it you don't go for this plan, because you start adding back carbohydrate as soon as blood sugars go down to normal.

VIRGINIA: I'll tell you why we don't recommend this kind of an extreme diet. It hearkens back to the old Atkins weight-loss diet or the so-called drinking man's diet of the 1960s. It was discovered that if someone consumes less than 60 grams of carbohydrate a day, they are in a state of ketosis. That means they're burning their own body fat to convert it to fuel. Of course, they lose weight. The problem is that they're eating gigantic hunks of meat, as much as they want, and that increases their health risks. It increases some of the same risks that diabetes itself does.

A low- or no-carbohydrate/high-protein diet is dangerous on a long-range basis because it is by default a high-fat diet. Protein and fat hang out together. They're inseparable buddies. With a high-fat diet you can get very high blood cholesterol and very high low-density lipoprotein levels, and both of these contribute to cardiovascular disease. Yet another risk with protein is that it's hard on the kidneys. Actually, any diet that eliminates major food groups is not a good solution for a lifetime.

We do not recommend that you adopt a diet that is extremely low in carbohydrate and low in calories for more than a few days, just long enough to get your blood sugar down. For many people, and I am one of them, if I do a Fast Fast to control my blood sugars, I get a high level of ketones and they make me crazy. Some people love it. They feel real good, with lots of energy. But it makes me so berserk I'm liable to go out and attack a wheat field. Many people don't tolerate it any better than I do. And ketones make your breath smell funny.

JUNE AND BARBARA: Many people newly diagnosed with diabetes are sent by their doctors to a dietitian. In our opinion, this is definitely the way to go. People think the dietitian will tell them to get off sugar forever, but instead the talk is mostly about fat. We also noticed that at the Presbyterian Diabetes Center you have a teaching manual that recommends the "low-fat lifestyle." Why is fat such a big deal for Type II diabetics?

VIRGINIA: You're right in noticing that fat is a big deal. In fact, it may be the biggest deal for the Type II-R's, whose bodies actually have a preference for fat as a fuel source. Nondiabetics normally use glucose as their fuel of preference. The glucose is shuttled into the muscle cells via the cells' receptors. Glucose is used strictly as fuel; fat goes into storage.

Now let's say you're a Type II-R and your muscle cell receptors don't work so well. They can't make use of the insulin to get the glucose into the cell. One thing Mother Nature did for us as a safety valve was give us the ability to use fatty acids as well as glucose for fuel. So when they can't get to the glucose, your muscles can use fatty acids as their fuel to keep going.

When you eat a meal with 50 percent of the calories from fat, here come the two fuels, fat and glucose, floating down the bloodstream to meet your muscles. The muscles would actually prefer the glucose, but what will they do if they can't get the glucose in? They grab the fat and use it as their fuel and leave the glucose floating around. That's why you end up with high blood sugar after a high-fat meal.

This is not the way it works in people who don't have diabetes. In a normal person fat goes straight into storage and doesn't raise the blood sugar. Fat is not sugar. It doesn't even convert to blood sugar except under extreme circumstances.

But the Type II-R diabetic has high blood sugar because his or her body used the fat for fuel instead of the glucose; the insulin level is high as well because the insulin couldn't be used up getting the glucose into the resistant cells. Now the insulin is going to store the glucose as fat. So into storage it goes, and the Type II-R gains more weight.

A recent article in the *Obesity Journal* (I was asked to be the centerfold but I declined) looked at a large number of people with and without diabetes and measured their body fat levels and then tracked their eating habits over a long period of time. The researchers noted two things. One, thin people and fat people eat about the same amount of calories (this was already a well-known fact). Two, thin people eat less than 30 percent of their calories as fat, and fat people eat more than 30 percent of their calories as fat. This is the big difference.

So can we cut our fat consumption to 10, 20, or 25 percent of our calories and lose weight? The jury is not in on this yet, but it is certainly looking like the way to go. For the person with diabetes, this is neither as easy nor as difficult as it sounds. If you cut the fat, you have to add carbohydrate in order to have enough calories. To prevent the high-carbohydrate diet from raising your blood glucose levels, you have to be careful to add lots of fiber, because fiber slows the entry of glucose into the blood and also makes you more sensitive to your own insulin. If in combination with a low-fat and high-fiber diet you also get plenty of exercise, you'll not only lose weight, but you'll be the healthiest you could ever be! This is what we at the Presbyterian Diabetes Center call the "low-fat lifestyle," and if it's beginning to sound familiar, it should. It is the recommendation for a healthy heart, cancer prevention, and good health in general.

We advise people not to think of this as a diet. People who go on diets go off diets. We ask our patients to go on a life. Eating less than 20 percent fat requires some fundamental changes, but if you give yourself plenty of the carbohydrates that you love, you'll feel great and not get into the "deprivation mode," a surefire way to blow your diet!

JUNE AND BARBARA: We think you're onto something, Virginia. Fat, not carbohydrate, is the real enemy. Avoiding fat is the cornerstone of the successful Pritikin weight-loss (and health-gain!) diet and of the newer Martin Katahn T-Factor diet. It's also basic in Dr. James Anderson's high-carbohydrate, high-fiber, low-fat diet (HCF diet), which allows only 9 percent calories as fat but so improves insulin sensitivity in Type II diabetics that in one study the diet resulted in 52 percent of overweight Type II's being taken off insulin completely. Need we say more?

Now tell us exactly how you follow a low-fat diet.

VIRGINIA: Get obsessed with fat! Look for it everywhere. Get a calorie and nutrient counter paperback at the bookstore and start looking at every label of every food product you consider buying. Any more than 5 grams of fat in a serving is probably too much. To find out how many grams of fat you can have, estimate your total daily calories—for example, 1,600. Now multiply by 20 percent to find out how many calories of fat you can have. This would be 320. Now divide those calories by 9 to determine the grams of fat you can have (each gram of fat has 9 calories). The answer is 36. (That's seven fat exchanges if you use the American Diabetes Association's exchange lists). Thirty-six grams of fat are plenty to keep you dietarily happy.

Look at breakfast for example. Skim milk has no fat. (I use 1/2 percent milk to avoid the transparent look of skim, but that's only 1 gram of fat per cup, whereas low-fat milk contains 5 grams a cup.) Cheerios (and many other cereals, hot or cold) are fat free. A banana is fat free. Hey, this is really easy . . . no problem.

Now how about lunch? You were going to eat macaroni and cheese? Think again. A typical serving (about twice the recommended amount) has 35 grams of fat—your whole day's supply! You really have to watch cheeses. In fact, most cheese recipes— you know, a little leftover this and that and cover it with about a cup of grated cheddar and voilà, a masterpiece—are high in fat. All those years we watched the Kraft show on Sunday nights and *believed* that cheese was health food. And now you find out it was all a lie! We should have known that anyone who would put a glop of mayonnaise on Jell-o would lie about cheese, too!

So what are some good choices for lunch? Try a baked potato topped with low-fat cottage cheese and chives. Tastes better than sour cream. How about pasta with a tomato and mushroom sauce with no meat? If you want meat, make it skinless chicken, fish, or a very small serving of lean red meat. You'll have to be very careful about eating meat. In many cases half the calories in a meat serving come from fat. Put another way, the quarter-pound hamburger patty (3 ounces cooked) has 10 to 15 grams of fat—and that's without cheese or mayonnaise.

Dinner? Well, you must be getting the idea by now. Just get out that fat gram counter and you'll be safe.

JUNE AND BARBARA: It's really important to have one of these fat gram counters and understand clearly where fat lurks in food. A lot of people just don't get it. During the 1992 Republican convention we heard a radio interview from a Houston barbecue place that was a favorite of then-President Bush since back when he was in the oil business in that city. Bush had stopped by to eat while he was in town for the convention. The interviewer asked the owner of the place what Bush had selected for his meal. She said that he had barbecued beef, barbecued ribs, and hot links with cole slaw. She said that normally he would have had baked beans instead of the cole slaw, but he had told her he was on a low-fat diet. Wowee! The only thing that might possibly have been low fat in that place were the baked beans—assuming they weren't loaded with bacon or ham.

To keep you from inadvertently living off the fat of the land, we'd like to suggest a few fat gram counters so you can run right out and buy one while you're fired up on the idea. There's a huge choice, but we'll only list the ones you're most likely to find in your local bookstore.

The Corinne T. Netzer Fat Gram Counter (Dell, $4.50)

The Fat Counter by Annette Natow and Jo-Ann Heslin (Pocket Books, $5.99)

The T-Factor Fat Gram Counter by Jamie Pope-Cordle and Martin Katahn (Norton, $2.50)

The Vest Pocket Fat Counter by Susan Podell (Doubleday, $2.99)

(Note: If you have trouble finding these, write to us at 5623 Matilija Ave., Van Nuys, CA 91401 and request a *Diabetic Reader,* where you'll find reviews, excerpts, and ordering information for important books on diabetes.)

Incidentally, do you consider this super low-fat diet also good for Type II-Ds like June? We certainly hope so because June's a confirmed fatophobe. She practically runs screaming from the room when she sees something that's deep-fried or full of cream, butter, cheese, or any other notoriously fat-laden product. It's as if she had been frightened in her crib by a can of lard and it marked her for life. Barbara, on the other hand, seems genetically programmed to like fat—or perhaps it's more environmental since she's from the Midwest. But for whatever reason, she naturally gravitates toward things like fried chicken and barbecued ribs and biscuits and gravy like grandmother used to make. June has been on the lean side all her life, while Barbara, like so many other American women, perpetually feels she should lose around 10 pounds. There's an obvious message here.

VIRGINIA: As far as the low-fat diet for Type II-D's, I think it's a great idea. After all, it's a healthy diet for everyone! The only difference is that people like June who are insulin deficient may find themselves getting low blood sugar throughout the day. This is because they'll probably be taking more insulin to cover all that extra glucose mobilized by eating such a high-carbohydrate diet. Some II-D's may also need help from their diabetes health professional in learning how to use Regular insulin a little more cleverly in order to cover those higher carbohydrate meals.

JUNE AND BARBARA: When you come right down to it, just how easy—or hard—is it for most people to follow such a low-fat diet?

VIRGINIA: Take it from one who's doing it: it's not easy to get out there and live in the real world on a really low-fat diet. Temptation is ubiquitous. The first rule of thumb is: if it's fried, forget it! Cheese is a real no-no. This is the most painful part for me. I love cheese! At home I use the fat-free or low-fat cheese slices (Kraft Free, Lite Line, and Alpine Lace are good ones) although they're a little salty for my taste, because I also cut down on salt. There are a few dishes that you need a little bit of cheese for, and these nonfat or low-fat varieties do the trick. They even melt nicely.

Another thing I really miss is mayonnaise. There are some good low-fat mayonnaises such as Lite Hellmans, which has half the fat of regular mayo, but even so it has 5 grams of fat per serving. Kraft makes a fat-free mayo, but as far as taste goes—yuck! I have discovered that I can buy some extremely low-fat dressings. I've found one with parmesan and garlic (boy, is that good!) and I use that mixed with tuna to make a tuna sandwich. On turkey or chicken sandwiches I use mustard, which is totally fat free.

How are you going to eat a potato without any fat on it? Besides low-fat cottage cheese with chives or green onion, try salsa. It gives the potato a really nice flavor.

JUNE AND BARBARA: It's one thing when you're at home and in total control of the situation, but how about when you eat out? Eating in a restaurant is the hardest part of any diet—especially a low-fat one. Maybe you could give us a few tips on how you handle that.

VIRGINIA: Well, living in New Mexico as I do, my favorite food when dining out is our wonderful New Mexican cuisine. A typical New Mexican food is enchiladas. They dip a tortilla in oil, then in chile (a sauce of red chile, not like Texas chili), they put cheese in it and fold it over, then they pour green chile over it and add more cheese—plenty of cheese. They also serve a lot of refried beans. The classic way to make refried beans is to start with pinto beans and add a cup or two of lard or bacon drippings.

My favorite restaurant, however, prepares their beans with no fat. They're nothing but cooked pinto beans mashed up. They taste just as good as the refried ones with all the fat—maybe even better since you feel so virtuous when you eat them. Of course, I don't order the enchiladas. I order off the à la carte menu and pick fat-free dishes. For instance, they have an excellent dish called Potatoes Garcia. It's just sliced potatoes cooked down until they're real soft, with cilantro and a touch of green chile added. Boy, are they good! No fat and wonderful flavor. I get a big tortilla and eat the beans and potatoes mixed up with a little green chile. Green chile sauce has little or no fat. You can be selective like this in any restaurant. When you order fish, ask them to grill or broil it and leave off the fat. Leave off the sauce, too. Most restaurants are happy to do that for you.

When I go into a restaurant and order a meal that includes a piece of meat that is much larger than I need, I know I'll eat it all if it's on my plate, so I ask my husband to split the entree with me. We each order our own potato and salad. That way I'll be quite satisfied with a serving of 2 or 3 ounces of meat.

JUNE AND BARBARA: We handle that too-large protein serving in a different way. We each order a full portion but take half of it home in a doggie bag. It's not too hard to resist the temptation to eat all of it if you know the leftovers will save you the trouble of shopping for and fixing a protein course at home the next night.

You can ask for doggie bags even in the best restaurants. We have a friend who is very socially prominent and has gone to the fanciest of private finishing schools. She now works as a volunteer at UCLA giving conversation classes to newly arrived foreign students. They ask her questions about experiences they've had that were confusing or upsetting to them. One Korean girl told our friend she was out to dinner with her boyfriend and at the end of the meal the waiter asked her if she wanted a doggie bag. She said, "I was so frightened! I didn't know what to say or do." Our friend explained what a doggie bag is and assured the student that she should never hesitate to ask for one because everybody does it and it's a perfectly correct thing to do. If she says it's okay, it must be!

VIRGINIA: Most of us have found that we must play lots of little games with ourselves to make our diets work. One trick is to focus on what you *can* have. And what you can have makes a wonderful life. You can feel good and you can have health. Don't focus on what it is you can't have, because that's a racket that will get you in trouble.

JUNE AND BARBARA: People who are genuine fatophobes like June, may want to know if it's OK to eliminate all fat in an individual meal.

VIRGINIA: It's very difficult to eliminate totally 100 percent of the fat, although it's not impossible. You'll find, though, that if you eat a fat free meal it's also probably virtually a protein-free meal and that means you'll get a pretty steep glucose rise after the meal. As I suggested previously, if you're on insulin, you can learn to cover the carbohydrate with your insulin dose. For most people the formula is one unit of regular insulin (fast acting) for each ten grams of carbohydrate. You can do that and then do a one-hour after-meal blood sugar reading to determine your own formula for covering food with insulin. Another tip when you're going to eat a high-carbo meal is to take the regular insulin at least 45 minutes before the meal so the insulin will peak with the food.

I would like to comment, though, that no one would want to eliminate fat entirely 100 percent of the time because there are some incredibly important vitamins that we get from fat. These are the so-called fat soluble vitamins A, D, E, and K. Vitamin E is very important for keeping our skin soft and wrinkle free (as if that were possible!). It's also important for healing and we wouldn't want to slow that down. If you eat a normal diet of a little bit of meat here and there, use some olive oil once in a while on a salad, and have some dairy products (skim milk is fortified with vitamin D), you'll be safe on these vitamins.

JUNE AND BARBARA: Jane Brody, health columnist for *The New York Times*, recently wrote a column about a new category of eating disorder, distinct from anorexia or bulimia and far more common than either of these. It's called "binge eating disorder," and accounts for a large proportion of seriously overweight Americans who repeatedly try to lose weight but fail. You've probably met hundreds of diabetics who fit this description. If binge eating disorder is their problem, they indulge in frequent, uncontrolled, and often hours-long eating episodes during which they may devour more than 2,000 calories. Psychologist Richard R. Rubin calls these "search and consume missions." Unlike people with bulimia, they do not attempt to purge their bodies of the excess calories by inducing vomiting or taking laxatives. They simply gain weight.

According to Dr. Robert L. Spitzer, who proposed that this disorder be included in the official manual of psychiatric diagnoses so that insurance would reimburse for its treatment, binge eaters tend to be depressed, anxious, or suffering other psychological disturbances much more than other people with comparable weight problems. Here are the criteria to identify the condition:

Recurrent episodes of binging and the sense that the eating is out of control.

Episodes occur at least twice a week on average, for six months or longer.

The behavior causes marked distress.

Binges involve at least three of these actions: eating much more rapidly than usual; eating to uncomfortable fullness; eating large amounts of food even when not hungry; eating alone out of embarrassment; feelings of disgust or guilt.

Unfortunately, going on a diet does not solve this problem; in fact, drastic dieting may trigger binging behavior. Overeaters Anonymous is a good form of group therapy for bingers. In fact, Dr. Spitzer's study found that 71 percent of participants in Overeaters Anonymous met his diagnostic criteria for binge eating disorder.

From your experience with seriously overweight diabetics, would you say that many of them have this psychological problem? If so, will treating it put them on the road to weight loss?

VIRGINIA: I'm sure that Dr. Spitzer is onto something here. I frequently encounter patients who use the very words, "My eating is out of control." There is one more stimulus that he hasn't noted that I feel may be very significant for a Type II-R. As you proceed down the merry path of Type II-R diabetes—highly insulin resistant, making excessive amounts of insulin to control your blood glucose, but even so, only partially controlling it—your blood glucose goes up incrementally. In other words, you can sort of control your blood glucose, but if it goes up due to a dietary indiscretion—such as if you "accidentally" ate a chocolate bunny for Easter—your body cannot bring it back down and you will stay at the higher level. This is the phenomenon we've called glucose toxicity. It is a condition where your insulin works better at normal range glucoses. It also takes a lot more insulin to conquer a high blood glucose than to maintain a normal range. Type I's and

Type II-D's will also notice this phenomena, but it is much more pronounced in Type II-R's.

JUNE AND BARBARA: June can certainly verify this. If her blood sugar is in the low 200s, it takes a supplement of only one unit of insulin to return her to normal blood glucose (90–100). But if she gets wildly out of control, say the high 200s or low 300s, it takes two units to get her back down to 200, plus a third unit to get her down to normal. She's lucky enough to be able to get back on track by injecting supplements of insulin, but as you point out, those Type II's who don't take insulin just stay up there.

VIRGINIA: That's why we do the Fast Fast. It brings blood glucose down quickly. You become more sensitive to your own insulin and if you keep your blood glucose normal for a while, often then you can control it by watching your diet and you'll be less likely to have hunger attacks.

One reason why many Type II-R's binge is the huge amount of insulin they're getting, especially when their blood glucose is out of control. As a Type II myself, I can "feel" an insulin rush during and after meals. It feels a little like the insulin reaction (blood glucose going too low) that Type I's get when they overdose on insulin. When I'm getting an insulin surge I feel my lips quiver, but when I look in the mirror they aren't moving. Sometimes I get a little quivery feeling in my chest or neck. This is why many Type II-R's will tell you that they aren't hungry all day—until they eat something. They get a rush of insulin with the food and that gives them the munchies. Then they proceed to eat all evening long. I'm sure that June can confirm this feeling. When you feel a surge of insulin in your body, it is very difficult not to eat something. I've found that if I can explain this reaction to people, they can live with it—and cope with it—better. For years they've probably been beating themselves up about having no willpower.

Besides these insulin surges that cause overeating, I feel that getting yourself into a "deprivation" mode can trigger the binge disorder; at least it does for me. That's why the 20 percent fat diet works so well. The fact that you don't limit your serving sizes on the good-for-you foods gives you the strength to avoid the bad stuff. We have a patient with Type II-R, a woman of 35 who has lost 30 pounds in the last four months. The other day she told me, "I can live like this forever, because I know I can have what I want when it comes to fruit, pasta, and veggies." I'm confident that she's going to be able to avoid the pitfall of the deprivation mode and binge eating.

JUNE AND BARBARA: In the recommended diets, sugar is a no-no but starch is OK. Why is this? Aren't they both carbohydrates?

VIRGINIA: As it turns out, there's very little difference. The biochemist calls starch a complex carbohydrate because it is a long chain of glucose molecules, as opposed to simple sugars that are made up of only a few glucose molecules. Our dietitian at the Presbyterian Diabetes Center, Beverly Spears, uses a great visual demonstration for this concept. She has several strings of those great big pop beads babies play with, which she has the patient break apart. Guess what? The long chain breaks apart just as easily as the short chain. This is the reason that the "glycemic index" studies found that white starches and white sugar are not very different in the effect they have on blood sugar. The glycemic index is a tool to measure the relative effect that different foods have on blood glucose. Different glycemic index studies have shown that white rice, mashed potatoes, and sugar have a similar effect on blood glucose. Does that mean that the person with diabetes should not eat potatoes or white rice? No, what it means is that you shouldn't eat a big bowl of white rice or mashed potatoes for a meal. A study reported in the *Diabetes Educator* (the journal of the American Association of Diabetes Educators) found that orange juice and Coca-Cola affect blood glucose exactly the same. What that means is that you should eat the whole piece of fruit instead of drinking juices. (Yes, I mean "no sugar added" juices as well; Mother Nature has already added the sugar.)

The sum total of all this is that a little sugar is not necessarily a problem for the person with diabetes. You can have goodies such as low-sugar cookies (animal cookies, vanilla wafers, gingersnaps, etc.), low-sugar cakes with no icing (Cool Whip makes a great cake or cupcake topping), or low-sugar frozen yogurt or ice creams.

JUNE AND BARBARA: We might mention here, too, that the American Diabetes Association is definitely in accord. They say it's OK to have up to one teaspoon of sugar per reasonable serving of food, and the maximum number of teaspoons you can have each day depends on your individual caloric needs. A lot of diabetes cookbooks also use small amounts of sugar in the recipes.

Getting back to the glycemic index, we're reprinting it below so that everyone can see that some complex carbohydrates are more complex than others and don't send blood sugar up as fast as mashed potatoes. In this group are things like apples, sweet potatoes, black-eyed peas, and all kinds of beans. These are the "slow" carbohydrates, the ones that should help you keep your blood sugar more stable. Incidentally, Virginia, they're the very foods you've been telling us we should make the largest part of our meals—cereals, pasta, veggies, whole fruit.

GLYCEMIC INDEX

This index compares the extent to which different carbohydrate foods raise blood sugar. Since glucose raises it the highest and fastest, it is assigned the index number of 100. The lower the number, the less impact the food has on raising blood glucose levels.

Simple Sugars

Fructose—20	Honey—87
Sucrose—59	Glucose—100

Fruits

Apples—39	Bananas—62
Oranges—40	Raisins—64
Orange Juice—46	

Starchy Vegetables

Sweet Potatoes—48	Instant Potatoes—80
Yams—51	Carrots—92
Beets—64	Parsnips—97
White Potatoes—70	

Dairy Products

Skim Milk—32	Ice Cream—36
Whole Milk—34	Yogurt—36

Legumes

Soybeans—15	Garbanzos—36
Lentils—29	Lima Beans—36
Kidney Beans—29	Baked Beans—40
Black-eyed Peas—33	Frozen Peas—51

Pasta, Corn, Rice, Bread

Whole-wheat Pasta—42	White Bread—69
White Pasta—50	Whole-wheat Bread—72
Sweet Corn—59	White Rice—72
Brown Rice—66	

Breakfast Cereals

Oatmeal—49	Shredded Wheat—67
All-Bran—51	Cornflakes—80
Swiss Muesli—66	

Miscellaneous

Peanuts—13	Sponge Cake—46
Sausages—28	Potato Chips—51
Fish Sticks—38	Mars Bars—68
Tomato Soup—38	

The big problem we've always found with the glycemic index is that it only analyzes a small selection of carbohydrate foods and that leaves the majority of carbohydrates out there in mysteryland. That's why many dietitians say you have to test out individual carbohydrates on yourself and see which ones cause you to have normal or abnormal blood sugar. In other words, you create your own glycemic index by checking your blood sugar level after eating a portion of a particular carbohydrate food. That way you can learn to predict the potential effect of foods on blood glucose and plan accordingly.

VIRGINIA: That reminds me that the glycemic index rates pasta as a good carbohydrate. I've had some patients say they can eat a lot of pasta and not have a problem, but others say it really raises their blood glucose. I think I know the answer. The more you cook your pasta, the more you make it quickly digestible. Boiling too long changes the starch of pasta to sugar. So you need to cook it *al dente* in the true Italian manner.

JUNE AND BARBARA: That's the way it tastes best, anyway. Now we need to know how long it takes different foods—protein and fat, as well as carbohydrate—to cause a rise in blood sugar.

VIRGINIA: Carbohydrate foods will cause a blood glucose peak about an hour after a meal. Only about 10 to 30 percent of the calories from protein convert to glucose, and they're released into the bloodstream over a period of 4 to 8 hours after a meal. Fats may or may not cause a blood glucose rise. In Type II-D's, they don't tend to cause an increase in glucose, but in Type II-R's, where the body doesn't use glucose very well, the cells tend to use fat as a fuel source more easily, and therefore the glucose from the meal tends to be increased in the bloodstream because it is not being used by muscle cells (our old friend insulin resistance is at work here).

What you need to do to get a reasonable rise in glucose after a meal is to eat a *balanced* meal—carbohydrate plus some protein plus some fat (less than 30 percent of calories in fat). Considering the above peaking schedule for different kinds of nutrients, we can get a good postmeal level if we add lots of fiber besides the protein and the fat. Don't get me wrong about protein. I'm not suggesting a high-protein diet. In fact, a low-protein diet is better for all of us.

You can plan on 1 ounce of protein at breakfast, 1 or 2 ounces at lunch, and 3 ounces at dinner. This is a fairly low-protein diet, but by including a little protein with each meal, lots of vegetables both raw and cooked, and starches with fiber (brown rice, baked potato with skin), you get a better glucose after meals; Type II-R's get improved utilization of glucose by increasing insulin sensitivity.

JUNE AND BARBARA: We've heard that when you're trying to lose weight, it's not a good idea to drink your calories. Liquids slip down too easily, and since you don't get any chewing satisfaction from them, you may feel hungry and go off and eat a bunch more calories in some more substantial form.

VIRGINIA: Yes, it's my philosophy never to drink calories. You can have so many good things like all those diet soft drinks that are calorie free, so why waste your calories on liquids? Also, liquid sugar absorbs so fast that you can't even cover it with insulin to get a decent blood sugar reading. We tell our patients to avoid all fruit juices and eat the fruit instead. Did you know that you have to smash eight apples to get just a half cup of juice, and then you've thrown away the best part—the fiber?

For people who are addicted to their juice in the morning, we suggest Crystal Lite's citrus blend flavor. It tastes like orange-pineapple juice and it has no calories. My personal favorite flavor is the pink grapefruit.

JUNE AND BARBARA: How do you feel about getting liquid calories via alcohol? We don't want to be accused of advocating drinking, but we feel it's our duty to acknowledge the big media blitz about the "French Paradox" of two glasses of red wine a day lowering cardiovascular risk and increasing HDL ("good" cholesterol). Not long after that revelation, we read in *Diabetes Care* (April 1992) about a new study from Bordeaux, France, which showed that two glasses of wine with a meal have no adverse effect on glycemic control in people with diabetes. In fact, there was a slower rise in glucose after the meal in non-insulin–dependent Type II's than if they had water with their meal instead of wine. So you'd better hurry up and tell us what's wrong with drinking before the French lead us down the wrong path.

VIRGINIA: A "lite" beer or glass of dry wine with a meal is no big deal, but if you do serious drinking, you'll probably find that it does serious damage to blood sugar control. You should never drink alcohol on an empty stomach because your liver gets preoccupied with the alcohol and forgets to put glucose back into the blood when your blood sugar starts getting low. That's why people on pills or insulin are always advised to have their drink with a snack or meal.

It's important to remember, though, that there are 7 calories per gram of alcohol, just 2 calories less than fat! A 3-ounce glass of dry wine has 70 calories. If weight is a problem, you need to take that into consideration before you start following the French Paradox prescription. And, of course, with hard liquor you should use only sugar-free mixes. Better still, use sugar-free mixes without the alcohol!

JUNE AND BARBARA: We've often heard from dietitians that Type I's need to count carbohydrates and Type II's need to count calories. Would it be true then that while Type II-R's should count calories, Type II-D's, who are presumably not overweight, would be better off counting carbohydrates the way Type I's do?

VIRGINIA: Yes, in fact we teach people who are learning to use Regular insulin to count carbohydrates so they'll know how much insulin they need to take to balance their blood sugar. As I said before, we use a formula of one unit of Regular insulin for each 10 grams of carbohydrate in order to get a good after-meal blood sugar. But it is important for each individual to test about an hour after a meal so they can determine their own insulin-to-carbohydrate formula.

Some Type II-D people use a basal-bolus insulin system. This means they take slow-acting insulin twice daily to cover their basic body functions and what health professionals call a bolus (a concentrated dose) of Regular insulin before each meal to cover the carbohydrate in the food in that meal. With practice they can get very talented at looking at a meal and assessing the carbohydrate content and calculating how much Regular insulin they need. Doing this enables them to get the best control. Of course, they would still want to look at their total diet for fat (in order to not get too much) and important nutrient elements (in order to get enough). Man and woman do not live by carbohydrate alone.

JUNE AND BARBARA: What about the so-called dietetic and diabetic foods? Of late we've noticed that there are mail-order food companies that handle nothing but special sugar-free sweets and treats for diabetics. Are they good for you and worth the usually inflated prices?

VIRGINIA: These candies, cookies, jams, and other items are usually made without sugar or their main enticement is that they're low calorie. I've heard our dietitian Bev's talk on these a number of times. She gives a lesson in label reading. When the label says "no sugar added" and you look at how the product is sweetened, it may be with concentrated fruit juice, or with something like corn syrup, which is not sugar but has the same effect on blood glucose. The number of calories will often be no different from regular food. We often see this in cookies, especially. Dietetic cookies may have 30 calories apiece, just like regular cookies and at twice the price. We recommend eating regular cookies that are low in fat and sugar, such as gingersnaps, vanilla wafers, animal cookies, or plain little shortbread cookies. Read the labels. Find a cookie that has less than 2 grams of fat for each serving (which may be from two to six cookies, depending on size). These are going to be much lower in price than dietetic varieties and cause little or no rise in blood sugar.

The other group of foods to watch out for are the dietetic candies. Most times these are sweetened with sorbitol, mannitol, or other substances with "ol" on the end. They all have a laxative-like effect. Hard candies or chocolates with mannitol or sorbitol as their sweetener will have fewer calories than regular sugar candies, because they are a little lower in fat. It's not the sugar that makes the difference, because sorbitol and mannitol sweeteners have about the same number of calories as sugar. But for some people a very little bit of this type of product causes severe gas cramps and possibly diarrhea. (The last thing you want to do on a long trip is give your child a pack of Velamints with sorbitol.) Sometimes caramel corn or other specialty products advertised for diabetics are also sorbitol sweetened. These "dietetic" products cost more, and we don't think they're worth it. We like to teach the person with diabetes to have a little bit of sweets containing a little bit of sugar. A little bit of sugar is no problem in a well-balanced diet. Shop in regular markets and buy regular foods, not what's in the special sections of dietetic foods.

One of the interesting tidbits Bev discovered is that good old New York-style cheesecake does not cause much of a glycemic rise. That's because it's all fat and very little sugar. Some of us can't tolerate the calories of eating cheesecake very often, but for those who don't have a weight problem and especially for pregnant gals, this is a great alternative to eating cake. For Thanksgiving they can have pumpkin cheesecake. For the baby shower or other special occasion, they can have a small piece of cheesecake and feel like they're having a really yummy dessert without raising their blood sugar much.

JUNE AND BARBARA: You've mentioned that fiber can slow down the rise in blood glucose after a meal. Dr. James Anderson, author of *Diabetes, A Practical New Guide to Healthy Living,* has long advocated a diet high in complex carbohydrate and fiber (HCF diet) for people with Type II diabetes. His maintenance diet for overweight diabetics calls for 50 grams of fiber a day for a 2,000-calorie plan. The American Diabetes Association recommends that the diet include up to 40 grams of fiber a day. Since most people when diagnosed with diabetes are probably eating only 10 or 11 grams of fiber a day, they're missing the benefits fiber can give them. And it's not all that easy to up the fiber in your diet.

VIRGINIA: To give you an idea of how difficult it is to get 50 grams of fiber, a serving of Grape Nuts (1/4 cup) has 4 grams of fiber, a serving of Cheerios has only 2 grams, and a serving of Rice Krispies has *no* fiber. You have to eat lots of vegetables, fruits, and beans to get 50 grams of fiber in your diet.

JUNE AND BARBARA: We compiled the chart below so that everyone can see some of the foods that are particularly high in fiber. By including some of these foods in your meals you can start building up to your 30, 40, or 50 grams a day.

HIGH-FIBER FOOD CHART

(Listed in Descending Order of Fiber Content)

	Serving Portion	Grams of Fiber
Beans and Peas		
Black-eyed peas	1/2 cup	12.4
Kidney beans, canned	1/2 cup	7.9
Pinto beans	1/2 cup	5.3
Split peas	1/2 cup	5.1
White beans	1/2 cup	5.0
Breads and Crackers		
Pumpernickel	1 slice	3.8
Triscuits	6	3.3
Wonder high-fiber wheat or white	1 slice	2.9
Cornbread, whole-ground	1 piece (78 grams)	2.7
Graham crackers (2½" square)	3	2.1
Cereals		
All Bran with extra fiber (Kellogg)	1/2 cup	14.0
Fiber One (General Mills)	1/2 cup	13.0
Raisin Bran (Post)	2/3 cup	6.0
40% Bran Flakes (Kellogg)	1/2 cup	5.0
Fruits		
Raspberries, fresh	1 cup	9.1
Blackberries, fresh	3/4 cup	6.7
Pear, fresh	1	5.0
Strawberries, fresh	1¼ cup	4.1
Prunes, dried	3 medium	4.0
Apricots, raw, with skin	4	3.5
Nectarine with skin	1	3.3
Orange, fresh	1	2.9
Apple with skin	1 small	2.8
Plums, fresh	2 medium	2.4
Grains		
Spaghetti, whole-wheat, cooked	1/2 cup	2.7
Rice, brown, cooked	1/2 cup	2.4
Popcorn, air-popped	3 cups	2.0
Vegetables		
Artichoke, cooked	1/2	7.6
Squash, winter, cooked	1/2 cup	3.6
Pumpkin, canned	3/4 cup	3.3
Asparagus, cooked	3/4 cup	3.1
Green beans, cooked	1/2 cup	2.8
Zucchini, cooked	1/2 cup	2.7
Broccoli, cooked	1/2 cup	2.4
Carrots, raw	1 medium	2.3

JUNE AND BARBARA: Try as you may, though, sometimes it just isn't possible to get up to that 50-gram level, especially if you eat a lot of meals out. We agree with dietitians who maintain that the very best way to get your fiber, as well as all your vitamins and minerals, is from the food you eat. But when you can't manage that, then a fiber supplement can help you get the amount of fiber you need. You have to be careful, though, to get one that doesn't contain sugar or too much carbohydrate or your blood sugar will go up instead of down.

Our old favorite supplement, Fiber Excel, is no longer being made, but we've found another that we like: Yerba Buena Daily Fiber Formula. Health food stores usually stock it, but if you can't find it, get in touch with us (5623 Matilija Ave., Van Nuys, CA 91401) and we'll help you track it down. Also please get in touch if you find another good fiber supplement so we can check it out and spread the word.

Since it does take a bit of effort to get more fiber into your diet, Virginia, maybe you could tell us why it's worth making that effort.

VIRGINIA: High fiber in the diet has lots of advantages. Not only does fiber slow down the rise in blood glucose after meals, but it improves carbohydrate metabolism and lowers cholesterol and triglycerides. As if that weren't enough, fiber may also contribute to lower blood pressure and it can enhance weight loss in fluffy people.

You should eat a wide range of foods to include both kinds of fiber: soluble, such as oats, legumes, and fruits and insoluble such as wheat products and bran. High-fiber foods are low in fat and are very filling. If you get filled up on these good foods, you're less hungry and won't be tempted by a stray candy bar. The person who decides to try the high-fiber route must build up to it gradually and also increase fluids in the diet dramatically. High-fiber diets have social consequences, as a diet high in fiber will cause gas.

As for the fiber supplementation, such as you recommend, it appears to provide benefit only if your diet is comprised of at least 50 percent of calories as carbohydrate.

JUNE AND BARBARA: What about dietary supplements of other kinds for Type II diabetes? Magazines and newspapers are always coming up with minerals and vitamins and even herbs that they claim will improve or even cure diabetes.

VIRGINIA: People with Type II diabetes should probably add a mineral supplement to their regimen that includes magnesium and chromium picolinate, as these have been found to increase insulin sensitivity in many people. Another supplement to add is Vitamin E. Vitamin E has recently been found to improve your lipid levels and decrease risk of heart attack. Also, ask your doctor about taking a small dose of aspirin daily to reduce the risk of heart disease. These are simple but really important areas to watch because cardiovascular disease is the major cause of death for us Type II's.

JUNE AND BARBARA: Since we like people with diabetes to have as much flexibility as possible in their lives, how about skipping meals if the circumstances—such as plane delays in travel—might make it hard to come up with the right food at the right time?

VIRGINIA: Yes, you can skip meals as long as you're not on insulin. If you take one of the oral agents, you might start feeling a little low if you don't eat. Usually you won't, though, because your body makes extra insulin only in response to meals. If you don't have a meal for it to respond to, it won't make the insulin.

While skipping a meal once in a while is possible, it's really not a great idea because you may get too hungry and overeat at the next meal. Our dietitians strongly advise our patients always to get up and have a nice high-fiber cereal breakfast even if they feel like sleeping in and skipping that meal. Then have lunch. If you get hungry in midafternoon, have a snack, something like fat-free yogurt—fruit yogurt that is sweetened with Nutrasweet tastes great and is under 100 calories. Low-fat cottage cheese makes a good snack, as do raw vegetables with low-fat ranch dressing. And, of course, fruit is the all-time great snack. They also strongly advise another snack at bedtime. The reason for all these meals and snacks is that by spreading your calories throughout the day, you're less likely to store as many of them as you do when you eat them all at once.

Let's say your total daily calorie intake is 1,800–2,000 calories. If you divide them into more frequent, smaller amounts, you'll be much more likely to use them as energy sources. If, on the other hand, you don't eat all day and then consume 2,000 calories at one meal, obviously your body can't make use of all that and actually stores a higher percentage of the calories.

JUNE AND BARBARA: We always recommend that you eat like a cat, not like a dog. The difference between the dining habits of these two favorite animal companions was brought home to us once when we were going to be out of town and wanted to leave some food for a neighborhood cat who always made it a habit to drop by for dinner—and sometimes breakfast and lunch! We got one of those cylindrical containers that you can fill up and as the cat eats, the food drops down into the feeding bowl. The feeder had a stern warning that it was to be used only for cats, never for dogs; if you used it with a dog death might result! We asked the pet shop clerk why death would result if a dog used it. Was it that he might get his head stuck in the container and suffocate? No. The problem with dogs is they don't know when to stop. If you put a whole container of food out, the dog will dive in and, as the clerk said, "eat himself into oblivion." A cat, on the other hand, will just take a few mouthfuls of food now and then throughout the day— and sometimes throughout the night. Seldom if ever do cats eat large quantities at once, dog style. This is why, although there are such things as fat cats, you see them much more seldom than you do fat dogs. Dog owners often have to put their pets on diets because with the dog's typical one-big-meal-a-day program, they store up too much fat.

VIRGINIA: Yes, fat storage can be a hazard for all creatures great and small. But for a Type II-R it's a big-time hazard. That's because what we're talking about is building more fat, and more fat means more insulin resistance, and more insulin resistance just compounds our problems.

You may say, "Yes, but I'm not hungry until I eat. Then after the first few bites, I almost go crazy with hunger and it's a struggle not to overeat. I don't want to go through that more times a day than I already do."

I understand that terrible hunger feeling from experience. It's part of the disease. Food gives you a big insulin surge that makes you ravenous. From my experience, though, I also know that if you spread your food over the day and eat something every three or four hours, you'll find that you're far more able to control your eating and maintain your weight than if you eat all of your day's calories at one gigantic meal.

CHAPTER 5

EMOTIONAL ASPECTS OF DIABETES: MY ENEMY/MY FRIEND

We remember well the day of Wednesday, July 29, 1992, because that was the day we picked up Mary, our new Scottish-Fold kitten. That day was made even more memorable by a report we heard on National Public Radio's "Morning Edition." It was the story of Larry Trapp, the Lincoln, Nebraska, Ku Klux Klan Grand Dragon and head of Nebraska's American Nazi Party. Trapp lost both of his legs in 1988 because of diabetes complications.

From childhood, Trapp's life had been consumed by hatred of all those who were different from him; Jews and blacks were his favorite hate targets. So it was only natural that when Cantor Michael Weiser and his family moved into Lincoln, Larry began a harassment campaign, calling them at all hours to deliver anti-Semitic threats such as, "You're going to be sorry you ever moved here, Jew boy," and putting cards in their mailbox saying things like, "The KKK is watching you, scum."

Understandably disturbed, the Weisers contacted friends and the police for help whenever these harassments occurred. But after a while, Michael and his wife, Julie, started examining their own feelings. They realized that they were the victims of hatred, yes, but they had also become haters themselves. They hated Larry Trapp.

This realization caused Michael Weiser to come to the personal decision that he was going to change. He was going to practice the love, understanding, and forgiveness that he preached in his sermons at the temple. Cantor Weiser says that in Judaism, "The highest thing that a human being can do is to make an enemy into a friend." But he acknowledged that most of us never do that. As he explains, "We have an enemy so we either avoid that enemy or we fight with that enemy."

He decided that the only solution to the enmity he felt toward Larry Trapp was to become friends with him. To make that happen, he launched his own harassment campaign against Trapp—a friendship harassment campaign. He began leaving messages on Trapp's answering machine that tried to point him in the direction of love rather than hate.

One day when Cantor Weiser was making one of his regular friendship harassment calls, Trapp picked up the phone and started shouting at him to stop calling. Weiser ignored the shouting and said simply and kindly, "I know you're disabled. Would you like a ride to the grocery store?"

Trapp was quiet for a while and then said, "No, but I thank you for asking."

A few nights later Trapp called Cantor Weiser and told him that he needed to talk. The cantor and his wife immediately went to Trapp's house. He confessed to them how lonely he was, and the Weisers stayed and talked with him for over four hours. Trapp later said he had never met anyone who showed such love and caring as they did. At the end of their evening together, Trapp symbolically removed the two swastika rings he was wearing and handed them to the Weisers, saying he didn't need them anymore.

A few months later, Trapp converted to Judaism. When his health worsened—he was dying of kidney

failure caused by the diabetes—Julie Weiser quit her
job in order to nurse him full time. During the last
months of his life, Trapp spent his time meeting with
people who were willing to rethink their racism, showing them how his life had changed for the better with
love and without hate.

This moving story illustrates the Judaic principle of
making an enemy into a friend. This is a principle that
we all can and should apply to our daily lives.

Think about your diabetes. It's only human nature to
regard it as an enemy that threatens and torments you
every moment of every day. But, instead of letting yourself be consumed by hatred, try to turn that enemy into
a friend, a friend that teaches you valuable lessons that
you might not be able to learn in any other way, a friend
that constantly pressures you to make changes for the
better in your life.

In an article in the *Los Angeles Times,* "Forever Set in
Your Ways at 30?" health writer Shari Roan reported
that studies show that by age 30 or 35, your personality
is pretty much set for the rest of your life. Major
changes are difficult to achieve and unlikely. There is,
however, an exception to this rule: "Catastrophic
events, such as developing a serious illness or losing a
loved one, can change people."

Ms. Roan cited the example of Mark, a rock band
singer who lived a wild and dangerous life that included
taking drugs. When a van in which Mark was riding
crashed, he was left paralyzed from the waist down.
Mark now considers this accident the best thing that
ever happened to him. It spurred him to get off drugs,
to go to college and on to graduate school, and then to
launch into a successful professional career. As he says,
"I don't think I would be here today if this hadn't have
happened."

In a study of people who had experienced significant
events in their lives, either positive or negative, psychologist Richard G. Tedeschi at the University of North
Carolina found that negative events are the ones most

likely to cause people to make changes. "Negative life events are so affecting that they call into question a lot of the usual ways of operating that people have adopted. Only because they're so traumatic do they pull people off their usual path."

Dr. Tedeschi goes on to say that people who have been transformed by negative events "often adopt a different philosophy of life . . . they begin to feel that life is good and useful; they become more expressive, more empathetic and tolerant."

The strangest revelation of this study is that profound *positive* events don't change people dramatically. This is because positive events don't challenge our basic ideas about living and what life is all about the way negative events do. In other words, unlikely though it may seem to you at the moment, diabetes can improve your life more than winning the lottery! It can, that is, if you neither avoid it nor fight it, but turn it into a friend.

We'll now ask Virginia to show you some of the emotional steps you can take to establish that friendship and make it a long-lasting one.

—June and Barbara

What You'll Find in This Chapter

Denial
Motivation
Attitude
Family and Friends
Stress
Sex
Fear of Insulin Injection
Adjusting to Loss of Spontaneity

JUNE AND BARBARA: We all know that people have different emotional reactions to a diagnosis of diabetes. Some have a healthy fear of what might happen to them, so they go to work on this diabetes thing. They get medical advice—and take it! They read, they go to support groups, and they take charge of their own health. They may become healthier than they were before they ever heard of diabetes. This group, unfortunately, is by far the minority.

What most people do at first—and this is a common strategy of self-protection when we feel overwhelmed—is simply deny the diagnosis. We hear the word "denial" a lot in modern life. "He's in denial" means that in order to function at all, the person must push whatever has happened that he doesn't like so far back in his mind that he doesn't even recognize its existence. For those of you who aren't familiar with denial, maybe this parable will illustrate what it's like.

THE PARABLE OF DENIAL

Once there was a man named George who deeply resented the fact that there was such a thing as gravity and that his life was so affected by it. He detested gravity from the very moment he first became aware of it when he was 5 years old. He was holding his mother's favorite antique bud vase. It slipped from his fingers and fell and shattered on the floor. He never forgot how upset his mother was.

He loathed the fact that snow and rain and hail and apples and everything else dropped down, never up or sideways. He hated tripping and falling and banging his knees—all because of that #$@%^&* gravity. George began to spend most of his time brooding about gravity and how it loused up what would otherwise have been a perfectly lovely world.

As time passed, his resentment got worse. He despised gravity and the restrictions it imposed upon him more and more until he finally could stand it no longer. He decided he was just going to ignore its existence. "I'm not going to let this gravity thing ruin *my* life," he announced.

From that day forward George pretended gravity wasn't there. If he held a piece of china or crystal in his hand, he let go of it and ignored the fact that it fell and broke. Before long his entire set of china and crystal was destroyed. He dropped his dachshund puppy so often that it would no longer come to him when he called. In fact, the puppy would hide when he came into the room.

Then, one day George was at work looking out the window of his office, which was on the twelfth floor. It was such a nice day that he decided he'd go for a stroll. He opened the window, stepped out, dropped 12 stories, and broke every bone in his body. He's now in traction in the hospital waiting for his bones to knit, with an elaborate pulley system holding up his limbs against the force of gravity.

The moral of this parable is that you can't change a situation with denial, and you'll only hurt yourself if you try.

Denial in reference to diabetes is a word we hear constantly from the lips of health professionals. So tell us, what is your secret of helping people overcome this formidable barrier to coping with and controlling diabetes?

VIRGINIA: I've just finished reading four Tony Hillerman books. They're wonderful stories about the Navajo people, and this question of denial reminds me of the Navajo word *horzo*. According to Hillerman, *horzo* is their term for being out of harmony. That's how I think most people feel when they experience the news that they have diabetes.

I rarely meet anyone who is totally surprised by the diagnosis. Usually they have had a suspicion, or else they have suspected they had something worse than diabetes. Nevertheless, when the diagnosis is confirmed there is almost always a period of grieving. The grief is often related to the losses that they anticipate diabetes will entail. Many times these are losses they have heard about or maybe seen in family members with diabetes: loss of freedom to eat what they want, loss of being able to schedule their time any way they feel like, loss of health or limbs or sight, even loss of life.

We approach each newly diagnosed person differently, depending on circumstances. For example, if the person is a pregnant lady, we cannot afford the time to work through the grief in a leisurely manner. We must get her blood glucose under control immediately. Because we're dealing with the health of her child, usually the patient can muster the spirit and energy to assist us with the task.

Many people, without the motivation of a pregnant woman, react with anger. They're angry at having diabetes and sometimes take it out on the health care practitioner who gives the news—

the old shoot-the-messenger strategy. Others simply won't accept the diagnosis. I've seen people go from doctor to doctor to doctor trying to get one of them to give a different diagnosis.

My approach is to support such people with care and information. I tell them that I have diabetes and have had it for 12 years. This usually helps them see that there is life after diagnosis. Then I try to give them information on how they will be able to live with diabetes day in and day out. I allow people to be unhappy about diabetes. Nobody has to like it, but we do have to go on living, and if you control your diabetes, you can live with it better and easier and healthier.

I encourage people to keep coming back for appointments at the Presbyterian Diabetes Center at least every two weeks until we see that they have a handle on the situation. We only work on survival skills for the first few months. People don't remember any of the complicated stuff if we try to teach it to them while they're still in a state of shock over the diagnosis. People look as if they're paying attention, may think they're on top of things, but if you ask them later what they remember about the first month or two after the diagnosis, often they can hardly remember a thing. This is true of many stressful events in people's lives. Can you remember the funeral of a close relative? Details of a divorce? We realize that the diabetes diagnosis is a traumatic event in their lives and try to give them only simple steps to follow.

How do I know this? When I was diagnosed with diabetes, I tried to approach it the way I do most things in my life: intellectually. "If I just find out everything about it, it won't affect me." Well, it affected me just like everyone else—with denial, grief, and depression. Because I know how they feel, I always try to encourage people to go easy on themselves for several months, to give themselves a chance to adjust to the diagnosis and to learn that living with diabetes is not as bad as they thought it would be.

After they've mastered the survival skills of diabetes (how to test blood sugar, take medication, and follow a simple diet), then we can move into the advanced course. We know when they're ready for this because they start asking questions. We also realize that we may have to repeat some of the information about survival skills at this time, because they were in a diagnosis trance the first time we told them.

Then we start them on our "In Charge" course. This is an eight-week, two-hours-each-week program where we give advanced lessons in living with diabetes: for example, how to eat out, how to adjust medications, how to prevent complications.

At the conclusion of this course, most people are ready to go to a schedule of visits to their doctor every three months plus checking in with diabetes educators from time to time for some fine-tuning. We find that many of our patients come in for a visit just to chat about how things are going and to find out if there is anything new in diabetes management technology that they need to know.

JUNE AND BARBARA: What do you do when you meet people with hard-core denial for whom your standard procedures don't work?

VIRGINIA: Yes, we sometimes meet people who can look at any evidence and only see what they want to see. For people like this, calling in family members or close friends may help. But sometimes we just have to wait them out and let them know how the disease is affecting them and give them plenty of space so they can come back for help and still save face.

There's one young man we see in our practice that took us six months to get in for diabetes education. He was diagnosed with Type II diabetes although he's only 36. He came to see one of our endocrinologists because his primary-care physician had sent him. He was a very busy business owner and was upset that these doctor visits took up so much time. His mother has diabetes and he knew exactly what to do without instruction—or so he thought. When he failed to keep his appointment with the Presbyterian Diabetes Center, we called and arranged a new one. He called and canceled. We arranged new appointments again and again. Again and again he canceled.

The way we finally got him to come in was by arranging the appointment with his wife, who realized the importance of good control. To make sure he got there, she came to the Center with him. Although it took many broken appointments to get him into the Center and out of denial and on track, he's finally getting into good control. His wife still comes with him to the appointments, and the two of them will be starting the "In Charge" class in two weeks.

JUNE AND BARBARA: Right up there with denial as a major emotional problem in diabetes is motivation: trying to make yourself do the things you know you should do for your diabetes and yourself. Usually denial is a one-time thing and once you get rid of it, it's gone forever. But that need to keep motivated is something you will always have to struggle with. Just how do you keep yourself motivated day after day, year after year, your whole life long?

VIRGINIA: That's a tough one! Almost every time I go to a diabetes conference for health professionals, there's a session on how to motivate your patients. The problem with diabetes is it's relentless. It's there day in and day out. It never goes away. It never lets up. If you get disgusted and decide that you'll just forget about it for a while, it will sneak up and whap you up the side of your head to remind you that it's still there.

JUNE AND BARBARA: Well, since it *is* always there and you *do* need to do all those day-in-and-day-out (boring!) things to take care of your disease, what can you do about making yourself keep on keeping on with it?

VIRGINIA: You need to get the right attitude about it. You probably think, "I'm sick and tired of fooling with this diabetes thing every day. I'm sick and tired of never taking a break from it." And yet if I were to ask you, "Aren't you sick and tired of having to eat and drink every day? Do you pick up a piece of fruit or a glass of iced tea and say, 'I just hate it that I have to keep putting these things into my mouth and swallowing them every day for the rest of my life!'" No, you generally don't complain about that. You don't complain that you have to go to the bathroom several times a day forever or that you have to brush your teeth after each meal. There are a lot of things that we have to do all the time that we don't complain about. That's where that right attitude comes in. We have to decide that our diabetes routines are a basic part of life like taking baths and sleeping and breathing and do them without getting all worked up about it. That way instead of being an odious chore, they become almost automatic and we can turn our thoughts to more pleasant things.

JUNE AND BARBARA: It also helps if, instead of grumbling and muttering about your odious chores and how deprived you feel and other disagreeable things, you focus on what's good about your life, the things that make you happy—in other words, develop more of an optimistic attitude.

VIRGINIA: That's my philosophy. I've always felt that taking a positive approach, seeing the glass as half full rather than half empty, seeing the doughnut rather than the hole, has been very important to my success in life.

But even though I'm generally very positive and optimistic, I have to admit there's one area in which I'm not. I'm a pessimist about optimism. That is to say, I'm not very optimistic that people who are very pessimistic will ever turn optimistic. In my experience people who see the glass as half empty and who only see the hole in the doughnut hardly ever change.

BARBARA AND JUNE: This reminds us of something we once read in an autobiographical novel by James Kirkwood, the author of *A Chorus Line*. The title of the novel, *There Must Be a Pony*, was from a story about twin boys. One was an incurable optimist; the other an incurable pessimist. Their father, who was trying to give each son a more balanced perspective on life, hit upon a scheme. On Christmas Eve he filled one room of the house with every toy and video game a boy could ever dream of having, and put a tag with the pessimist's name on the door. He filled another room from floor to ceiling with equine excrement and put the optimist's name on that door. The next morning he told the boys where to find their presents. An hour later he came back to see how each had reacted to his gift.

The pessimist was sitting on the floor in the midst of all his toys, sobbing and wailing and miserable because he couldn't decide which toy to play with first. The optimist was laughing and singing and whistling, merrily shoveling all the equine excrement.

"What's going on here?" asked the father. "Why are you so happy?"

"Gee, Dad," replied the son, "I figure that there must be a pony here somewhere."

Optimists we don't really want to change. It's the pessimists we'd like to do a little attitude adjustment with. Why do you figure it's so hard to get them to change?

VIRGINIA: Maybe it's because there's no motivation for them to change because they keep proving themselves right all the time, and that gives them a kind of perverse satisfaction. The militant pessimist will also tell you that he's never disappointed. He thinks of himself as a realist and regards those of us who are very positive and who see things optimistically as perfect fools.

But the thing about being optimistic and seeing things in life positively is that you often prove yourself right. When I look back on my life I see that almost everything has turned out positively. I am where I am because of how things evolved, and I am happy where I am. How can I—or anybody else—say I'm not in the right place?

Once when I was introducing myself to a class and telling them that I had Type II diabetes, a patient in the front row looked up at me and said, "Well, how do you like it so far?" And you know how you tell the truth when you're not really thinking about it? I looked at him and said, "Well, actually it's been a tremendous professional advantage." It's true. To me diabetes has been a positive experience in many ways.

JUNE AND BARBARA: To us, too! We wouldn't have had half the experiences we've enjoyed and met one-hundredth of the wonderful people we now know—including Virginia!—without diabetes. We know of many people for whom diabetes has had a positive impact—people who wouldn't have become doctors or nurses or dietitians or exercise therapists or psychologists if they hadn't had diabetes and been determined to learn more about their disease and to help others. We even know two young women who found the loves of their lives through diabetes. One was a diabetes teaching nurse who met her husband when he was the representative of one of the meter companies who was calling on her hospital. The other love story is a bit more complicated. The woman had diabetes and it inspired her brother to invent the Medicool, which keeps insulin cool when you travel, hike, drive in the car, etc., and even keeps it warm if you're off in the snow. (Come to think of it, this is a double diabetes positive—a successful business and true love!) At any rate, the woman and her brother had a booth at a medical trade show to demonstrate the Medicool. Working in the booth next to theirs was the president of a company making another medical product. Between exhibit hours, they all got to talking and the upshot is that she's now engaged to the booth neighbor.

We're so fascinated with how-diabetes-brought-me-happiness stories that we're collecting them. If you come up with such a positive tale, we hope you'll write to us and tell us about it. We'll publish it in *The Diabetic Reader* so everyone can have their spirits lifted. (Write to us at 5623 Matilija Ave., Van Nuys, CA 91401 to tell us your story or to request a *Diabetic Reader.*)

But it's not just people with diabetes who need to have a positive approach and a spirit of optimism. Their friends and family members need that attitude, too.

VIRGINIA: A good example of this is Cathy Feste, who is a diabetes educator as well as a person with diabetes. She tells the story about what happened when she was a child and was in the hospital just after being diagnosed. She asked her mother, "What does it mean that I have diabetes?"

Her mother said, "It means that our family will all learn to eat better and we will all be healthier." We should all be so lucky as to have family members who take that kind of approach. It really rubs off onto the person with diabetes. All diabetes educators are inspired by Cathy's positive approach to managing diabetes both for herself and for her patients.

But still it remains a challenge for diabetes educators to take a person who is very depressed or who sees diabetes as a tremendous burden and turn this attitude inside-out into a positive one. And it's an even greater challenge for the person him- or herself.

It's funny how life gives us gifts that we can use positively or negatively. It makes me think of my friend Marci Draheim from Cedar Rapids, Iowa. Marci is a wonderful diabetes educator who also is an accomplished musician. She writes and arranges her own music and uses the power of music to help people experience their emotions in a positive way. She expresses her feelings about helping people with diabetes with a beautiful ballad she composed, called "I'll Be Here for You." She is a perfect example of a person using the gifts God gave her to help others.

JUNE AND BARBARA: Is there any way to effect an attitude change in depressed and negative people and get them to start using their own natural gifts in a positive way?

VIRGINIA: It's no secret that helping other people is a key to helping yourself. I encourage my patients to get involved in the American Diabetes Association or the Juvenile Diabetes Foundation as volunteers. When you're working with other people and trying to help them, it's much more difficult to focus on how miserable you are yourself. So get involved, if not with diabetes, then with some other organization that interests you. Focus on doing something positive for other people. I guarantee it will drive a lot of the negative out of your own life.

Finally, I have to say to discouraged diabetics: Lighten up and don't be so serious about it. Maybe right now diabetes is on the front page of the newspaper of your life. It's not something that will ever get out of the news, but it can certainly be moved back to the lifestyle section or maybe even the comics page. It certainly doesn't need to be forever printed in bold front-page headlines like "BOMB EXPLODES!" or "WORLD COMES TO AN END!"

JUNE AND BARBARA: It's often said that diabetes is a family disease in the sense that it has an impact on the entire family, not just the person who has it. Just what goes on in families when diabetes raises its ugly head?

VIRGINIA: The way I put it is: People don't have diabetes; families have diabetes. Diabetes affects the entire family and may change the relationships and communication patterns among all family members. Family members may experience the same fears and anxieties as the person with diabetes—sometimes even more intensely. To add to that negative, the diabetic may feel as though he or she has a "low position" in the family and has no right to expect family support or assistance with diabetic routines or crises. Conversely, the diabetic may feel a role diminishment or power dilution if the rest of the family is handing out advice and instruction on his or her daily activities.

The situation grows even worse when the diabetic person decides to keep the disease private and not allow any family participation in order to protect the family from the stresses of diabetes. Or the person with diabetes may not allow the other members any involvement by simply ignoring the hazards of out-of-control diabetes and doing nothing much to manage it. If the family and the diabetic have an unspoken pact to ignore diabetes management, they become "coconspirators" in the diabetes denial racket. This is often displayed by the nondiabetic members encouraging the diabetic to go off the prescribed diet with tempting goodies or planning activities that make it difficult or impossible to stay on the regimen. Diabetics will participate in this racket, because it's then possible for them to temporarily allay nagging thoughts about their inability to participate in activities like other people. It's as if they think they can avoid feeling the pain and fear of complications and possible loss of life. But in fact diabetes cannot be ignored. Denial of fears and failure to communicate feelings just cause more stress and emotional pain for everyone concerned.

I can't emphasize too strongly the fact that enlisting your family members in active participation with diabetes management is the first step to good control.

JUNE AND BARBARA: That may not be easy to do. We've seen husbands and wives really irritated because one or the other has diabetes. Sometimes they resent diabetes and all the expense and trouble it can cause. One spouse can be extremely critical because the other cannot seem to handle diabetes well. Occasionally we've witnessed loud family arguments over aspects of diabetes, real knock-down-drag-outs in public. So how do you go about creating good, positive family involvement?

VIRGINIA: There are several important steps.

1. Give your family permission to participate in your diabetes management. This is the step most often neglected and the pri-

mary reason people don't receive support. Sharing your life together means sharing the difficulties as well as the joys. Invite other family members to participate in diabetes activities such as support groups, education classes, diabetes association meetings. Remember that an invitation can be accepted or declined. Do not be judgmental about this.

2. Openly communicate your feelings. All members of the family must have the opportunity to express their fears and anxieties about diabetes, its complications, the restrictions of diabetes management, and especially their feelings about activities they may find repugnant, such as blood glucose monitoring or shots. Just getting people to express their feelings openly helps diminish the impact of those feelings.

3. Everyone in the family needs to learn the principles of diabetes management in order to give effective support. The whole family needs to get as much education about diabetes as possible. Each person needs a realistic understanding of what to expect from diabetes and what to do to ensure the best possible outcome.

4. You can make everything more comfortable for everyone, including yourself, by accepting diabetes rather than denying it. If you can't accept your diabetes, you'll find it difficult to accept support from others. Being in a position of dis-ease with diabetes leads to a constant feeling of not being OK, so your self-concept is diminished. Acknowledge that you're an OK person, a good person, and that diabetes is not a reflection of who you are. If you have a feeling of being at fault about having diabetes, this guilt and anguish will color all your relationships and interactions with others.

5. Listen to love! You should actively translate the comments and suggestions about your diabetes management made to you by your family members as expressions of love and caring. That's what they are. If your family didn't care about you, they wouldn't bother to comment on your diabetes activities at all. You can transform your relationships by reinterpreting what may have appeared to you as annoying criticisms into what such comments truly are: expressions of love and concern.

This is what any psychologist will tell you, and I know it to be true.

JUNE AND BARBARA: It's impossible, as you know, to talk about feelings and emotions without talking about stress. And stress, as any experienced diabetic knows, can play havoc with blood sugar. June was once stunned when she found out that facing a particularly worrisome situation caused her blood sugar to shoot up from around 100 to over 200 in less than 15 minutes.

VIRGINIA: I could write an entire chapter on stress and diabetes, because it's such a knockout punch to blood sugar control.

JUNE AND BARBARA: Why don't you start out by defining stress so we'll all be perfectly clear on what it is?

VIRGINIA: Stress is any change in your environment that causes the body to activate its stress response and release stress hormones. These hormones are meant to rev up your energy so you can fight or run from the threat. This is the well-known "fight or flight" response to danger that is left over from primitive times when there were all those lions and tigers out there, not to mention lots of club-wielding two-footed enemies. What happens is the adrenal glands are alerted and they cause the release of glucagon (the opposite hormone from insulin; it raises blood sugar). Glucagon in turn signals the liver to release its stored glucose. This extra glucose is what causes the problem for us diabetics, because we can't make enough insulin to match the highly increased glucose levels. That's why June's blood sugar shot up like that. Her injected insulin wasn't enough to cover the extra glucose triggered by the unanticipated stressful event.

JUNE AND BARBARA: What kinds of events and emotions cause this "fight or flight" response?

VIRGINIA: Both physical stresses and emotional stresses activate the response. Illness, pain, infections, injuries, surgery, pregnancy—all these physical stresses raise blood glucose because of the release of stress hormones in the body. Probably more common in our daily lives, though, are the emotional stressors like work pressure, family problems, fights with your mate, money difficulties, hurricanes and earthquakes, and the endless upsets and crises people face in modern life.

JUNE AND BARBARA: Some people seem to be under *constant* stress because they have a lawsuit pending, or are in the midst of a divorce or child custody fight, or are trying to care for an elderly parent and take care of their children at the same time, and so on. We have found, too, that diabetes itself causes plenty of stress in most people's lives. Wouldn't you agree that diabetes is another constant stress?

VIRGINIA: I couldn't agree more. Ordinary events that aren't stressful for nondiabetics become major emergencies for the person with diabetes—things like, "Dinner will be late this evening," or "Your suitcase hasn't arrived with the rest of the plane's luggage." At any moment of the day you can find something that interferes with what you're supposed to be doing for your diabetes at that particular time. Tests showing high blood sugars can generate all kinds of fear: fear of blindness, kidney failure, or foot amputation. Not having the money to afford the test strips causes stress. I could go on and on. That's why at the Presbyterian Diabetes Center we teach our patients about the damaging effects of stress and how to change their response to it by stress management strategies.

JUNE AND BARBARA: Ever since we wised up about stress and its effects on health we've been working on ways to handle it. In fact, our *The Diabetic's Total Health Book* is full of stress-reducing techniques, from exercise and meditation and visualization to such far-out methods as pets, travel, laughter, and hugs. Let's hear your antistress ideas, Virginia, as life in the '90s looks as if it's going to feature new and weird stresses that we've never encountered before. We all need to be acquainted with every form of stress therapy that's been invented—and then some.

VIRGINIA: I'm glad you realize you can't avoid stress, and therefore the more you practice the management strategies that work for you, the better. Here are my ideas on how to help yourself come to grips with stress:

Reduce the frequency of stressful incidents.

1. Make changes in family, social, and work commitments. Find activities that provide pride of accomplishment and satisfaction.

2. Set attainable goals and reasonable expectations so that disappointments do not become major stress points.

3. If you take insulin, learn to adjust your diabetes regimen and lifestyle so that the likelihood of severe insulin reactions is lessened; always carry glucose tablets and snacks.

Reduce the intensity of the stress response.

1. Learn Conscious Relaxation and practice it regularly (See the Conscious Relaxation exercise that follows).

2. Use meditation or prayer.

3. Decrease consumption of stimulants such as caffeine and nicotine.

Increase physical activity.

1. Exercise reduces stress by relaxing muscle tension and increasing cardiovascular function.

Focus your energy.

1. Identify the areas in your life that consistently result in frustration.

2. Control what can be controlled, and accept what can't be controlled. Remember, it's easier to ride a horse in the direction it's going.

3. Take action! Set your priorities. List tasks and break them into manageable sizes. Be realistic and flexible about time frames to achieve your goals.

CONSCIOUS RELAXATION EXERCISE

Practice this exercise in a comfortable place with little likelihood of interruption. If you fall asleep doing the exercise, as some people do, plan for awakening, if you're doing this on a short time frame (such as a lunch break at work). Get into a comfortable seated or lying position without crossing your arms or legs. Read over the exercise and then do it for yourself, using a similar scenario, or read it onto a tape and play the tape back. You may want to put your favorite relaxing music on the tape as well. Similar types of relaxation exercises are available on commercially recorded tapes.

Start this exercise by taking a deep breath . . . and letting it out very slowly. Feel the tension going out with the air. Throughout your busy day, deep breathing can be a quick and effective relaxation exercise. Put a small dot of colored tape on your clock at work and let it be a reminder to you that every time you look at the clock you will take two deep breaths.

Take another deep breath and as you let the air out slowly, allow your eyelids to gently close. Feel your body settle into your chair and get very comfortable where you're sitting or lying. Now you will begin relaxing by talking to the muscles of your body and allowing them to get completely relaxed. Start at your head. Feel the muscles of your scalp getting very relaxed. Your head will begin to feel warm and relaxed and your forehead will relax. Notice that your face is relaxing and smoothing out as you feel the tension leaving your muscles. Notice the relaxed warm feeling moving around to the back of your head and neck and your head is feeling heavy and relaxed. Allow your head to sink deeper into your pillow or chair or to fall forward on your chest as your neck muscles lose all tension. Feel a warm flow of relaxation moving all around your neck into your shoulders and notice your shoulders drop as all effort leaves the muscles.

Now take another deep breath as you allow all tension to leave your head, neck, and shoulder area. Feel the wave of relaxation moving down your arms as all tension in the muscles of your upper arm, lower arm, and hands now flows out through your fingertips. Your arms are now completely relaxed and feel warm and heavy. Feel the warm, relaxed feeling moving across your chest and into your back. You can feel the tension leaving all the muscles of your back and abdomen as you sink deeper into your chair. Now allow that warm wave of relaxation to move through your lower back and buttocks and into your thighs. Feel a wave of relaxation moving into your legs as all tension leaves the muscles and flows through your knees, lower legs, and ankles. All tension and effort is now leaving your body through your toes, leaving the muscles completely relaxed and warm.

Now take another very deep breath and as the air flows out feel a final wave of warm relaxation wash over your body from head to toe, removing any tension left in any muscles. Now we will get into a deeper level of relaxation by counting down to the deepest level of relaxation. You will get more and more relaxed with each count as we count from 10 down to 1. You will hear the cue words "calm and relaxed" often. These will be your cues so that at any time, any place, you can return to this same level of relaxation by saying to yourself "calm and relaxed" and taking two deep breaths.

As we begin the count, imagine yourself on a beautiful, warm day with the sun shining in a blue sky. You are lying on a thick, fluffy cloud. You are completely supported, your body is totally comfortable and relaxed. Feel the gentle rocking of this beautiful white cloud as it gently floats you toward your most favorite spot on earth. Begin floating downward as we count 10 . . . calm and relaxed . . . 9 . . . you are floating gently toward your perfect place . . . 8 . . . calm and relaxed, deeper and deeper . . . 7 . . . feel the warmth and gentle rocking of your cloud . . . 6 . . . calm and relaxed . . . 5 . . . you are floating toward the place you most enjoy being, it can be a real place or a place you have only imagined . . . 4 . . . calm and relaxed . . . 3 . . . sinking deeper and deeper into relaxation . . . 2 . . . see your favorite spot . . . you are more relaxed than you have ever been . . . 1 . . . you are completely calm and relaxed . . . your cloud has brought you gently to your perfect place . . . look around . . . you can see in detail how beautiful this place is. Look at yourself in this picture . . . notice how relaxed and healthy you look in your perfect spot . . . take a deep breath and say to yourself . . . "calm and relaxed" and know that you can return to this feeling of calmness and relaxation at any time by taking two deep breaths and saying to yourself "calm and relaxed."

Look at yourself in this picture and see yourself as healthy and happy and solving any problems you may have. You are now in a state of complete calm, health, and happiness. As you watch yourself in the picture you can see yourself getting healthier, handling all your day-to-day concerns with ease and grace. You can see that this feeling of relaxation will stay with you throughout your day. You will now leave your special place but your feeling of well-being and relaxation will stay with you and you will feel refreshed and full of energy. You will become more and more alert as we count from 1 to 4 and you will be fully awake, alert, and relaxed and feeling wonderful . . . 1 . . . 2 . . . 3 . . . 4 . . . welcome back.

JUNE AND BARBARA: Although this is as much a physiological issue as a psychological one, this might be as good a place as any to discuss sexual problems sometimes associated with diabetes since they can have such an emotional impact on all concerned. Breaking with tradition, let's put the gentlemen first. Does Type II diabetes cause impotence?

VIRGINIA: I hate to be the bearer of bad tidings, but yes, it can. Studies have reported that up to 50 percent of diabetic men over the age of 50 have some degree of impotence. In fact, after many other symptoms of diabetes have been ignored, impotence is sometimes the symptom that finally drives men to the doctor where they're first diagnosed as diabetic.

The primary physiological cause of this is neuropathy (nerve damage). The nerves that serve the penis and are responsible for erection become damaged by many, many years of high blood sugar. This causes an inability to achieve and maintain an erection. As with the other complications of diabetes, maintaining normal blood sugars can prevent this. Naturally, it's best to prevent it, since it is understandably very upsetting to a man. His libido is still intact, but he is unable to perform sexually. This can be extremely distressing not just for a man, but for the woman in his life as well.

JUNE AND BARBARA: What should a man do when confronted with impotence?

VIRGINIA: The first step is to have an evaluation by a urologist because there can be other reasons besides diabetic neuropathy for impotence and erection difficulties. If, after all the tests are done, the urologist ascertains that diabetes is the culprit and the problem is physiological, not psychological, there are some very good ways to help with this problem.

Among the best are the vacuum erection devices. With these, a tube is place over the penis and air is removed to create a vacuum. The vacuum simply pulls blood into the penis and causes erection. These devices are not very expensive, don't require surgery, and have been helpful to many couples. The cost is often covered by medical insurance, including Medicare.

Another system that some people have found effective is to use injections of a drug such as papaverine or phentolamine that will cause blood to be pulled into the penis and cause erection.

Some people resolve the problem with surgical implants, either inflatable or semirigid. Although some men and their wives have found these to be very effective, some serious complaints have been reported about them. Sometimes additional surgery has been required to replace defective implants or to remove them entirely or to repair the damage they have caused. A penile implant is something that you should investigate thoroughly and not enter into lightly. The best thing you can do is to talk to several men who have had one and see how it worked for them and what problems they encountered.

JUNE AND BARBARA: Now it's the women's turn. Do they also have diabetes-induced sexual problems?

VIRGINIA: Yes, although they're much less common, or at least they're less obvious and less frequently reported. It also may be that women's sexual problems are taken somewhat less seriously by the predominately male medical researchers. On top of that, most doctors may not be as careful about asking their women diabetes patients about sexual problems as they are about asking men. In a commentary in the Vol. 4, no. 1 issue of *Diabetes Spectrum* by L. A. Bernhard, Ph.D., R.N., it was reported that in a survey of physician members of the Diabetes Association of Greater Cleveland, 85 percent of those who responded said they routinely asked diabetic men about sexual difficulties, but only 33 percent routinely asked women.

Another article in that issue of *Diabetes Spectrum,* "The Differential Impact of Diabetes Type on Female Sexuality," described a study that made a surprising finding. Type I diabetes was found to have little effect on sexual responsiveness and sexual relationships in women. On the other hand, Type II diabetes had "a consistently deleterious effect on both the women's sexual behavior and their sexual relationships." The Type II women "viewed themselves as less sexually attractive, were less happy and satisfied with their sexual partner and sex life in general, were less interested in and more likely to avoid sexual activity with their spouse, and were less likely to lubricate adequately and to reach orgasm. . . . Their sexual activity was less varied and, understandably, they developed dyspareunia (discomfort during intercourse) more frequently."

JUNE AND BARBARA: And to think that people always consider Type I diabetes the more serious and restrictive and devastating condition! Were any reasons given for this bad news for Type II women?

VIRGINIA: The researchers had a number of theories. One was that Type II women may experience more of the autonomic neuropathy that prevents adequate lubrication. (The autonomic nerves are the ones that control the heart and blood vessel muscles and the glands.) Another was that Type II diabetes may have a more negative effect psychologically and socially because it generally occurs later in a woman's life than Type I and disrupts long-established relationships. The husband has often been the center of attention in the marriage, and when the focus changes to the wife's diabetes, a certain amount of marital conflict results. On top of that, a Type II woman sometimes experiences mood disturbances, especially heightened anxiety and depression that may decrease her emotional availability to her spouse. Still another hypothesis is that because Type II diabetes usually happens at middle age or later and is often accompanied by a weight problem, some of the sexual problems may have to do with a negative self-image, which in turn is caused more by the problem of over-weight than by diabetes itself.

But before any of you Type II women let yourselves get all bent out of shape over this research and start overanalyzing yourself and possibly creating sexual problems that weren't there before, remember that this study was of a total of only 55 women (32 Type I's and 23 Type II's) and certain aspects of the findings were in conflict with findings in other equally reputable studies. But most important, remember that as Dr. Bernhard said in her commentary on the study, "each woman is first an individual with her own personal characteristics, and she may not be anything like the group (type I or type II) to which she belongs."

JUNE AND BARBARA: Clearly if the woman sees that her problem is a psychological one related to diminished self-esteem, then some kind of psychological counseling would be in order. But what if it turns out to be more a physical problem caused by that autonomic neuropathy you mentioned?

VIRGINIA: Fortunately this kind of neuropathy is not as common as peripheral neuropathy—the kind that causes pain and eventual numbness in the feet and legs—but still it can be quite troublesome to the diabetic woman, especially when it interferes with her sexual function or enjoyment. There are creams and jellies, such as the KY brand, that can aid the lubrication problem. As far as the autonomic neuropathy itself is concerned, the only treatment we can offer at the moment is the ever-popular, all-time favorite diabetes panacea: *get your blood sugars in control!* There are some medications on the horizon (not yet available) that may eventually help with all kinds of neuropathy. They are called aldose reductase inhibitors. It's nice to be able to look forward to these, but still nothing beats that well-controlled blood sugar when it comes to combating neuropathy.

JUNE AND BARBARA: Of all the intense emotions that assail people with diabetes, especially Type II's, one of the greatest is fear of having to taking insulin injections someday. Since insulin therapy is the last resort for treating Type II diabetes and many

Type II's never have to take insulin, people can have months or years or even a whole lifetime to live with the dread of "going on the needle," as it's often called. They build up a fear that is totally out of proportion to reality. We should know because June experienced that fear for a whole year while she was trying to make it on diet and pills.

Of course, certain individuals actually have a true pathological terror of needles, known as needle phobia among psychologists. What words of comfort do you have for all those people out there living in various states of dread at the thought of taking insulin injections?

VIRGINIA: Many of us who have diabetes and have taken insulin can tell you that it is the least of the issues of having diabetes. As far as we can see, the biggest issue is not about having to take insulin but about not getting to eat brownies. This deserves far more attention and correction than all the emotion and upset surrounding insulin.

Still, I have seen patients who avoid going to the doctor, avoid participating in their own health care, and try to deny their diabetes altogether over the issue of taking a shot of insulin. Granted, taking shots is not everybody's favorite thing to do. If you have been avoiding the doctor out of fear that he or she might say you have to take insulin to get in better control, let me tell you this is one of the biggest nondeals in America today. The insulin syringes are 29-gauge needles. That's about the diameter of a hair. Ninety-nine percent of the time, with good technique, you literally can't feel them going in and out of your tummy. (Tummies are definitely the best place to give insulin.) So having to use insulin is not an excuse for not being in good control.

One thing we point out to people all the time is that giving an insulin shot, if it hurts at all, hurts a whole lot less than sticking your finger to check your blood sugar. You want to get out there and find the needles that hurt the least and check out the special devices for shooting in the needle. (The effect of these is to give you perfect injection technique.) Try out all the new technology and take advantage of the goodies you find to make insulin injection easier.

I have a lot of patients who say they wish they'd gone on insulin much earlier, because they feel so much better after getting their sugars under control. This improvement in the way they feel overcomes the minor inconvenience of having to give injections twice a day and drives fear of injecting right out the door.

JUNE AND BARBARA: Over the years when you talk to people who are discouraged about the things they've lost in life—or *think* they've lost in life because of diabetes—what seems to bother them the most?

VIRGINIA: Although they may tell about it in different ways, it all boils down to just one loss, the only real loss: the loss of spontaneity. That's the ability to do what you want to when you want to do it on the spur of the moment without having to plan ahead and make special arrangements. It can be as simple as spontaneously deciding you'd like to go out to eat in a restaurant and order whatever you feel like at the moment. Or it can be a little more complex, like something I observed a few weeks ago.

I was doing a diabetes program for a hospital in Midland, Texas. We all had a great time, but since it went on all day it was quite strenuous, and I was looking forward to getting a little rest on the one-hour flight to Albuquerque. But the plane had some seats that faced each other, unlike the usual airplane seating where everyone is facing forward and you can catch a little nap if you feel like it. Just my luck, I got one of those seats and a couple plopped down across from me.

This lady was bound and determined that we were going to talk. I mean, she was the original Chatty Cathy. She delighted in telling me that up until 30 minutes ago they had no plans to go to Las Vegas. (The plane was going on to Las Vegas from Albuquerque.) They just got home from work and suddenly decided, "Hey, let's go to Las Vegas for a couple of days."

"So here I am!" she said. "I don't even have any clothes with me. I didn't even have time to put any makeup on." She'd brought her makeup with her and proceeded to put it on right there in the plane. They planned to buy some clothes when they got to Las Vegas. These people had the money, the freedom, and the spontaneity in their life to do that sort of thing. We should all be so lucky to be in the oil business (pronounced "awl bidness" in my part of the country) so we could do just that—if we didn't have diabetes, that is.

Your limitation as a person with diabetes is that you can't just hop in the car, run to the airport, jump on a plane, and go to Las Vegas. No, you'd have to plan your supplies and your injections and your meals. But then, how many of us can jump on planes on the spur of the moment anyway? We have jobs, families, and responsibilities that keep us tied down to a routine. Diabetes can actually be a positive factor to get us organized and stay in touch with reality if we let it.

JUNE AND BARBARA: Yes, it's true, diabetes can organize your life better than any of those books or courses on how to bring order out of your chaotic existence. But if spontaneity is the biggest thing in your life, you can be spontaneous if you plan for it. That sounds like a contradiction in terms, but it really isn't.

People are always telling you to be prepared for any emergency. We're especially conscious of this in California with our earthquakes, but other states have things like tornadoes and hurricanes and floods. You need to be prepared with a kit containing all your diabetes supplies and snacks so you can pick it up and run if disaster hits. We once heard David Marero, Ph.D., a psychologist from Indiana University, speak on being prepared. His theory was, why just be prepared for terrible happenings? The same preparation works for wonderful happenings as well.

Suppose someone says to you, "I want to take you on a horseback ride up into the hills and we'll have a picnic supper and listen to music and watch the sunset." Do you say, "Oh, drat! I can't go. I don't have my insulin (or pills or whatever)"? No, you say, "Terrific. I'll just grab my Spontaneous Happy Event Kit, and we're off."

We know a young diabetic guy who practices what you might call modified spontaneity. He and a buddy pack their bags and his diabetes supplies and they go to the airport and take the next plane that's going somewhere no more than an hour or two away. His diabetes never causes him any problems—at least no more than it would at home.

So you see, spontaneity is possible. But, really, we've found that in the modern world, spontaneity is becoming an overrated commodity. Before June's diabetes diagnosis, we used to travel in Europe by buying a Eurailpass and jumping on a train—any train—and getting off wherever the mood struck us. Then we'd wander around until we found a hotel room. No more. And that's not just because of diabetes. More and more people are traveling, and the hotel you decided to stay in is likely to be *"complet"* as the French say or "fully booked" as the British put it. Ditto for the restaurant you'd like to eat in. If you want to have a really great trip, you need to plan it as carefully as a space launch. That's what we do now, and guess what! It's a lot more fun than winging it. You get weeks and weeks of anticipation as you prowl through guidebooks picking out where you want to visit, corresponding with picturesque hotels in convenient locations, even reserving special restaurants ahead of time. By the time you get there you feel you know the place, and that knowledge sets you free to relax and enjoy yourself.

So if you prefer spontaneity or anticipation or a combination of the two, you can have it in most areas of your life. Diabetes won't stop you. We don't need to envy the "awl bidness" pair—except maybe for their money!

PAYING THE BILL FOR DIABETES: DOLLARS AND NONSENSE

Dealing with the financial aspects of American medical care these days is like walking into a madhouse, and it's beginning to seem like the most violent shock treatments are reserved for people with diabetes. Your first problem is getting health insurance at all, because insurance companies are only willing to insure perfect specimens. It's like the automobile insurance companies wanting to insure only people who've never had an accident and are statistically unlikely to have one.

It's not so bad if you live in California, Colorado, Connecticut, Florida, Georgia, Illinois, Indiana, Iowa, Louisiana, Maine, Minnesota, Mississippi, Missouri, Montana, Nebraska, New Mexico, North Dakota, Oregon, South Carolina, Tennessee, Texas, Utah, Washington (State), Wisconsin, or Wyoming. These states either already have pooled-risk insurance programs or soon will because of laws passed by the legislatures. Any insurance company that wants to do business in one of these states has to contribute to a fund that will issue health insurance to those who would otherwise not be able to obtain it or would only be able to get it for exorbitant rates. (A portion of the pooled-risk funding may also come from state revenues.) They cannot charge more for pooled-risk insurance than 125–150 per-

cent of the average health insurance premium in that
state.

But let's say you don't live in one of those states.
That's when the craziness begins. An article in the *Los
Angeles Times,* "Working Without a Net," described what
happened to a self-employed man with the preexisting
condition of diabetes. When he quit his previous job to
start his own business, the cost of private health insurance for himself and his wife started doubling every
three months. When it hit $16,000 a year—just about
equal to the amount of his annual income—he had to
shut down his business and go to work for a government
agency just to get the medical insurance to cover his diabetes.

The article also told of growing numbers of people
who are hanging onto jobs they've outgrown or detest,
simply to keep their health insurance. It's not only bad
for business to have all these unhappy (and therefore
less efficient) employees, but it takes all the joy and
enthusiasm out of the work life of the employee who is
being held a hostage to health insurance.

Even if you like your work and have insurance, your
situation still isn't totally sensible and sane. Each year
you find your coverage eroding and your deductible and
copayment increasing. This is because medical charges
are getting out of hand and out of sight. (The *Times* article gave the example of a woman who had a miscarriage
and ended up with a $6,000 bill for one night's stay in the
hospital. The bill included such charges as $14 for 4
ounces of mouthwash and $17 for a 15-cent sanitary
pad.)

And the underlying reason for such exorbitant
charges is the essence of nuttiness. Only around one-
fourth of hospital patients have private health insurance.
Therefore these people pay not only for their own care
but for a portion of the care of those who have no coverage and those who have Medicare or Medicaid, whose
payments, set by the government, are not adequate by

hospital standards. This makes about as much sense as if you went to a restaurant for dinner and when you got your check, you discovered you were being charged to cover meals for three other diners who didn't have enough money to pay the bill.

Insane though the rest of the health-care system may be, Medicare is pure bedlam. June feels that one of the luckiest circumstances of her life is that she worked for a school district that had its own retirement plan, so she never contributed to Social Security. Therefore, she is not eligible for Medicare and remains covered by a private insurance plan, which, although it is not perfect, compared to Medicare is a thing of beauty (and rationality!) and a joy forever.

If you have Medicare, you don't need us to tell you how goofy it is. But if you're "looking forward" to going onto Medicare, try these on for size. Medicare will not cover your meter and strips unless you're on insulin— and even then your doctor has to fill out a questionnaire indicating that you're wildly out of control and heading for trouble. (In other words, you get rewarded with a meter and strips for not handling your diabetes well.) Then, even when your meter and strips are covered, Medicare never, under any circumstances, pays for insulin and syringes. In other words, it may pay for the things that show how your blood sugar is doing, but not for the things that are absolutely necessary to keep your blood sugar in control.

We could go on and on spelling out the problems with health care. But better that we do as Barbara used to when we were directors of the SugarFree Centers. If we were going out of town, she always left a list of phone numbers where we could be reached, so that others could "get in touch with us with the solutions to any problems that may have developed in our absence." So we'll ask Virginia to get in touch with you with solutions to the problems associated with the financial aspects of diabetes.

—June and Barbara

What You'll Find in This Chapter

Medicare
HMOs
Generic Drugs
Private Insurance
Pooled-Risk and COBRA Insurance
Medigap and Senior Plans

JUNE AND BARBARA: It would help if you could start with an overview of the kind of health insurance plans that are available, so we can understand what each has to offer.

VIRGINIA: It's important for everyone to understand the different types of insurance, but it's vital for people with diabetes.

Many people have an insurance plan that gives them the option of choosing an HMO (health maintenance organization). For people who have a chronic disease like diabetes, these plans have some advantages and some disadvantages. One advantage is that if you require lots of medications, these programs usually allow you to get them for a nominal copayment (the amount you have to pay out of pocket) of $5–$10 for each prescription. A disadvantage is that they often operate under a formulary. This means that they have a committee that selects medications for their plan. They make their selections based on effectiveness and price. To achieve cost savings they will select one or two specific drugs from each classification instead of allowing physicians on their plan to prescribe a variety of brand names.

For people with diabetes this means that you may not get your usual brand of insulin. This is one area in which I see many patients make a mistake. As long as you're receiving human insulin, there's probably no difference between brands and you should get whatever costs less. I've seen patients pay an extra filling fee just to get the particular brand of insulin they've been using. This can turn out to cost more than if they'd just forgotten about their HMO pharmacy service and gone out and bought the insulin retail.

Another way diabetics can cause themselves problems is when it comes to buying syringes. Let's say you prefer a certain brand of syringe, yet the HMO will only give you a lesser quality syringe for your copayment, and you think you're stuck (?!) with that. In fact, syringes are so inexpensive (especially if you shop around and find specials on them, and double especially if you reuse them four or five times) that you can buy them outside your copayment plan.

Where your copayment arrangement comes in handy is for expensive medications like those for high blood pressure. Those can be purchased with great savings on your prescription card.

JUNE AND BARBARA: This works well sometimes when you aren't even on an HMO. Barbara's mother, who has Blue Shield, can get her "maintenance" prescriptions for only $10 each if she buys them through a certain drugstore's mail-order plan. Of course, they prefer to give generics in this case, but if her physician insists, they will provide the exact drug prescribed.

We should mention some of the differences between generic and trade-name drugs. One of the best explanations we've seen is from Mike Voelker, Pharm. D., pharmacist at N.M.C. Homecare in Southern California.

"Generic drugs (drugs not protected by trademark) are in demand today and for many valid reasons. First, insurance companies and other health cost payment systems are encouraging their members to use generic drugs by offering people a lower copayment if they do. Second, the FDA (Food and Drug Administration) is shortening the time period for trade-name drugs to become generic. And, third, over the next three to four years the federal government is phasing in Medicare payments for prescription drugs, and just as many states do with their Medicaid programs, the federal government will probably demand that generic medications be provided whenever possible.

"For the above reasons it is safe to say that generics are here to stay. But, buyer, beware! Some warnings are in order. Brand-name drugs and their generic forms are not necessarily identical. Switching to a generic without proper precautions may cause serious problems. To understand the possible difficulties, you have to understand what generic drugs are and how they're made.

"A generic drug has exactly the same amount of the active ingredient as the trade-name product. The active ingredient by weight, however, makes up only a fraction of the total weight of the tablet or capsule. For example, a Lanatoxin 0.25-mg tablet weighs about 2.5 mg, but the active ingredient, digoxin, makes up only about 10 percent of the total weight of the tablet. The other 90 percent is comprised of what pharmacists call 'excipients'— fillers, binding agents, coloring, etc. It is these extra ingredients that very often determine how much of the active drug is absorbed into the bloodstream and how quickly. In some cases, more drug is absorbed with the generic form, and in other cases less is absorbed. This difference can be very critical, depending on the type of drug.

"With the following classes of drugs you, your doctor, and your pharmacist must be extremely careful when changing to the generic form:

1. Cardiovascular drugs (Lanoxin, Altace, etc.)

2. Hormone and related drugs (Premarin, Synthroid, etc.)

3. Psychotherapeutic drugs (Thorazine, Elavil, etc.)

4. Anticonvulsants (Dilantin, Depakene, etc.)

5. Oral hypoglycemics (Orinase, Diabeta, Micronase, etc.)

"A diabetic, for example, can switch from the trade name Orinase to the generic tolbutamide, but you should always ask your physician first. When the switch is made, you must be very diligent about testing for hyper- or hypoglycemia so that you can determine whether the generic is being absorbed in the same way as the trade-name pill. Then, once you have successfully switched, you have to make sure that you are always provided with that particular brand of generic because the same generics manufactured by different companies also differ in their excipients. This is another complication which means that only those in the know can protect themselves from drug overdose or underdose.

"With classes of drugs *not* on the above list, such as antibiotics and analgesics, it is perfectly OK to switch to a generic brand without any special monitoring.

"The final word on generics, then, is to enjoy the savings they offer, but make sure that you and your physician and your pharmacist work as a team to ensure their safe and efficacious use."

Incidentally, Voelker also told us that pharmacies actually make a greater percentage of profit on generics than on brand names, so if a pharmacist discourages you from purchasing a certain generic, he is doing so for medical reasons and not out of some sordid profit motive.

But let's get off drugs and back to HMOs. What else do we need to know about them?

VIRGINIA: Another significant feature is that they use a "gate-keeper" system.

JUNE AND BARBARA: What does that mean? Do they have someone guarding the door who won't let you in unless you can prove you're really sick?

VIRGINIA: It sounds that way, but it's actually a system that requires you to select a primary-care physician (a family doctor or internist). This physician will have to write you a referral before you can go to see a specialist.

BARBARA AND JUNE: Does this mean that you can't just march in and say, "I have diabetes and I want to see an endocrinologist"?

VIRGINIA: That's right. And you can't go directly to an orthopedist when you have a back problem, or to a psychiatrist if you're feeling depressed, and so forth. The reason the HMOs do this is so that the specialists won't be used indiscriminately when a primary-care doctor could have done as good a job. This makes sense. After all, patients aren't always adept at diagnosing their conditions and knowing what kind of specialist—if any—they need. It's also a cost-effective way of providing health care; but if you have a chronic disease like diabetes, it can become a hassle.

BARBARA AND JUNE: It certainly can. We've talked to lots of people with diabetes who belong to HMOs. They know from experience when they need to see an endocrinologist for a diabetes problem, and yet they're slowed down by having to first see the primary-care physician and then wait for him or her to decide that the problem truly is something that requires an endocrinologist's attention, and then wait to get the appointment with the endocrinologist. All the while, the diabetes problem goes untreated. Is there nothing that a diabetic can do to keep this situation from occurring over and over again?

VIRGINIA: Many HMOs in our area allow an endocrinologist to become a primary-care physician for individuals who have an endocrine disease. You should investigate and see if you can work out that kind of arrangement, because it gives you the best of both worlds: the care you need from your endocrinologist or diabetes specialist without the hassles of having to get a referral every time you need to see him or her.

One more thing you need to investigate when choosing an HMO: look into what they cover. Do they cover your blood glucose meter and strips? The strips are probably the most expensive part of diabetes management.

BARBARA AND JUNE: That certainly is something to look into! We knew of one young woman who was furious because her HMO wouldn't cover her meter and strips. Yet they would cover them for older people on Medicare (those who took insulin), because these people had signed their Medicare benefits over to the HMO and Medicare did cover meters and strips for them. The young woman resented the fact that she, who had a whole lifetime of diabetes ahead of her, was not provided with what was necessary to keep her disease in control, while the older people who had less risk of developing complications were. Obviously, it was more a matter of economics than concern for the well-being of the patient.

Another thing we have noticed about HMOs is that what is covered is often based on what kind of policy you have. Some people say, "I belong to SpendthriftCare HMO so I'll automatically get everything covered." Others lament, "I belong to SkinflintCare and they never cover anything." In many HMOs, some members may have a policy that covers no meters, strips, or prescriptions at all. Others have to pay a portion of the cost. And some lucky devils in the same HMO get virtually everything free of charge. The kind of policy you have, of course, is based on what your employer (or you as an individual subscriber) pays.

If you don't choose an HMO or don't have the opportunity to choose one, what are your other insurance options?

VIRGINIA: You could choose a standard indemnity-type insurance plan. This is traditional private insurance. This insurance covers a portion—usually 80 percent—of the costs of hospitalizations and outpatient services such as physicians and prescriptions after you meet a certain deductible. The downside of this kind of policy is that most of the time you must pay cash up front and then get reimbursed, so it can lead to a lot of paperwork.

JUNE AND BARBARA: We once read of a survey that revealed that the thing patients fear most about going to the hospital is not death, but the paperwork they're going to have to handle. We may be cynics, but we suspect that most insurance companies make filing for claims so difficult and keep bouncing back your claims for little niggling details so that you'll become so frustrated and discouraged that you'll just give up and they won't have to pay. Ernest Hemingway once said that if you want to be a writer, you have to be the world's most persistent son-of-a-bitch. The same thing holds true if you want to collect on your insurance.

VIRGINIA: There is an upside, though. With this kind of insurance you have complete choice about the care you get and the physicians and hospitals who give it to you.

JUNE AND BARBARA: But even this kind of policy, which we both have, is starting to "suggest" that you go to certain hospitals and physicians. They have contracted with these providers for a lower rate and the result is "a lower out-of-pocket expense to you." We always try to follow their "suggestion," but even so the "out-of-pocket expense" doesn't seem all that low.

VIRGINIA: That's because of cost shifting, which you touched on in the introduction to this chapter. Since it's referred to so frequently by health professionals and legislators when they talk about the crisis in health care in this country, let me explain in a little more detail what cost shifting is and, more important, why it exists.

Your doctor or pharmacy or other specialist is receiving reimbursement from a variety of sources such as Medicaid, Medicare, HMOs, PPOs (preferred provider organizations), indemnity insurance, and that small category of people who just pay cash. When the doctor receives payment from Medicaid or Medicare, it's been discounted greatly. If his fee for an office visit is $60, he may be getting only $20 from Medicaid for that same visit. The local HMO may be paying him only $35. If you have indemnity insurance you pay the full $60. Of course, you receive $48 back (80 percent of the $60), but only after you've met your deductible. The patient in the waiting room of an HMO will pay maybe $8 or $10 in copayment for the visit.

In the past, indemnity insurance was the preferred way to go. But more and more patients with indemnity plans are discovering that physicians and health-care organizations have to increase their fees to them to compensate for the discounting that's taking place on the other plans—thus you have the term cost shifting.

This cost shifting is getting to the point that the indemnity-insured patient is having to pay a higher and higher percentage of the total cost of health care. Those of us who have indemnity plans or pay cash are subsidizing Medicaid and Medicare by more than just our tax dollars. We're subsidizing it every time we go to the doctor or hospital.

Am I saying this cost shifting and subsidizing is good or bad? Neither. I'm just saying that this is how it is. Do I think we need a national health care system? Personally, I don't. When I look at current models of national health care such as the Veterans Administration, military hospitals, Indian Health Service, and the health-care systems in Europe, Scandinavia, and Canada, I don't see any of those systems that I would want to personally participate in. Would I send my child to the VA for health care? I don't think I would. I'm not saying that the VA doesn't have health-care professionals who work hard and care deeply about their patients. What I am saying is that their system is very inefficient and doesn't provide the level of quality care that I would like to see.

JUNE AND BARBARA: But don't you think we need some kind of improvement in our health care system? More and more people—often those with chronic conditions like diabetes—are falling through the cracks and getting no care at all, or else are going bankrupt from paying exorbitant medical costs, losing their homes, and then finally getting public assistance so they can have at least some kind of medical care.

VIRGINIA: I agree that we need something, but first we have to do a much better job with our public health care. It would take so little money, just the cost of one or two heart transplants in every state, to pay for the immunizations that could save a zillion lives. If the money from three or four amputations a year were put into the cost of shoes for people with at-risk feet, it could save the rest of the amputations.

America's health-care priorities need to change. We need to put more money, effort, and concern into preventing disease, into taking care of the basics extremely well—basics like prenatal care, immunizations, and the prevention of chronic diseases.

No, I don't want to see a national health care system like the much-praised one in Canada, where a person must wait two or three years to get gallbladder surgery because it's considered "elective."

JUNE AND BARBARA: It's true that the other systems aren't perfect, and we would want America to do a better job. But can we? Good medical care takes money—more and more every day—and there is less and less of that commodity available in this country.

VIRGINIA: Let me give you an example of how it can be done. At the Presbyterian Diabetes Center we have a pregnancy program where we work with women who have gestational diabetes and who have diabetic pregnancies. We have a team approach, where we involve the perinatologist (a doctor who specializes in high-risk pregnancies), the endocrinologist, and the nurses and dietitians in the Diabetes Center. We are able to manage these patients very effectively and monitor them closely and thereby prevent many problems of the diabetic pregnancy. We have normal-weight babies, healthy babies, babies who do not spend time in the Neonatal Intensive Care Unit. Yet with all that we are extremely cost effective. And that's not even considering the long-range cost difference between delivering a healthy baby and an unhealthy one.

JUNE AND BARBARA: But can this be done in a public health care situation?

VIRGINIA: Right now we're working with the Medicaid department in our state, trying to partner with them to help them do a better job of managing their patients in a cost-effective way.

That American Diabetes Association Recognition of Diabetes Education Centers Program I mentioned in Chapter 2 provides a way for third-party payers to know where quality care is being given and to be able to utilize resources more effectively so we get better care at a lower cost.

I think you may see in the future that the third-party payer— whether private insurance or public—will select for you the place where you will go for a certain surgery, the place you will go for your diabetes education, the places where you will go for other specialty kinds of care.

JUNE AND BARBARA: If you have health insurance, but you don't feel that it gives you the kind of coverage you want, is there any alternative or, because you have diabetes, are you pretty much stuck with what you have?

VIRGINIA: First off, you should remember that it's unlikely that you'll ever be totally delighted with your insurance coverage. No one has been since back in the days when some unions were able to negotiate contracts that included 100 percent coverage with no deductible. Those days are gone forever!

If you have pooled-risk insurance in your state, you could look into that to see if it's better than the insurance you currently have. To find out about this, call your local diabetes association or your state insurance commission and ask how to contact the pooled-risk insurance program in your state. Even if your state wasn't listed in the introduction to this chapter as having pooled risk, make these calls anyway. Pooled risk may have come to your state after this book was published.

But I must caution you to investigate very carefully and make certain you can get something else before you give up any insurance coverage. As previously mentioned, many people—especially people with diabetes—will find that they must select or hold onto a job simply for the insurance coverage that it offers.

Even if you're offered a different job that has good insurance and you would prefer to take the new job, you may wind up hanging onto the job you already have because the health insurance with the new company won't cover a "preexisting condition" for the first six months or a year or, in some dismal cases, as long as two years. If you have diabetes, this means your new insurance will be of little value to you during the preexisting condition exclusion period. After all, any health problem that you are likely to have may well be related to diabetes—or the insurance companies will claim that it is.

JUNE AND BARBARA: We've heard that if a company desperately wants to hire you, you may be able to negotiate a deal with them to pay for your extra coverage during this preexisting condition exclusion period. As Virginia says, though, know what you're getting into before you make any job changes, and, of course, make certain all promises are in writing.

But then, what do you do if the insurance change is not by your choice? What if you get caught in a merger or some other corporate upheaval and get laid off? Are you just left hanging out to dry?

VIRGINIA: No, at least not at first. You can take advantage of the government's COBRA plan. Despite the venomous sound of the name, it can be a lifesaver. COBRA stands for Consolidated Omnibus Budget Reconciliation Act, which, I realize, doesn't explain anything about it. What this plan does is give you the right to keep the insurance from your previous employer for up to 18 months. The bad news is you have to pay the premium yourself. The good news is that if during this 18-month period you have an accident or require surgery with a long recuperation period, the insurance company is obligated to keep covering you until the condition is cleared up.

JUNE AND BARBARA: What if you get laid off and join a new company that has a one-year preexisting condition exclusion? Can you use the COBRA until the preexisting condition period is over?

VIRGINIA: Unfortunately not. The COBRA plan is only for people who have no other health insurance at all. You can't decide to use it just because your new health insurance excludes your diabetes. I agree that if you have diabetes and your insurance doesn't cover diabetes, it's just about the same thing as not having insurance. But, snake-in-the-grass that it is, COBRA doesn't see it that way. This is just one more demonstration of the craziness of insurance coverage.

JUNE AND BARBARA: A lot of people who are on Medicare buy some kind of so-called Medigap insurance to try to plug up the holes in their Medicare. How does this work—or *does* it work?

VIRGINIA: The Feds have fine-tuned their regulations on Medigap plans. They fall into closely defined designations and the company must clearly indicate which plan the customer is getting. Some Medigap plans may cover only the copayment on Medicare-covered benefits. Other Medigap plans may cover expenses not covered under Medicare. Another option is an HMO that will take your Medicare contract for payment. You see these advertised as "senior plans."

The advantage to senior plans is that you get doctor visits and prescriptions for just a small copayment and no paperwork. The disadvantage is that you probably won't get as much choice about your physician. These programs must run very efficiently to make ends meet and therefore they usually offer no-frills care, but that doesn't necessarily mean poor quality. Many times they use nurses for triaging patients in their initial visit, to determine medical priorities and make sure they get the correct level of care. Often patients find that they actually prefer getting care from nurses rather than physicians because the nurses do more teaching and spend more time with the patient.

I guess our challenge for the future is how to get Cadillac care for Volkswagen prices. Actually, now that I think about it, Cadillacs and Volkswagens are both about gone. I guess our health-care system is going to have to become something like a Toyota: efficient, attractive, and moderately priced with excellent quality.

AT MY AGE, WHY SHOULD I BOTHER?

Now that we've come to the end of the questions on Type II diabetes, we're left with just one question—the one we've heard more than any other from people who are diagnosed diabetic in their adult years. This question is : "At my age, why should I bother making all these changes?" More specifically, "At my age, why should I start a whole new way of eating? I like the way I've always eaten." Or, "At my age, why should I start exercising? I've never liked exercise. I didn't like it when I was younger and I like it even less now." Or, "At my age, why should I try to lose weight? It's not easy—I should know because I've tried to do it dozens of times, and the weight never stays off anyway." Or, "At my age, why should I stick my fingers and take all those blood sugars? It doesn't feel good and it's expensive." And, finally, "What possible good can doing all these things do me at my age?"

We agree. If you're an oldie, you definitely shouldn't bother. It's a waste of time and it probably won't do you any good at all. Your next question might logically be, at exactly what age do you become an oldie?

That's not an easy one to answer. We've seen oldies who were in their 20s and 30s, and we've seen people in their 90s who were definitely not oldies. June started using the term "oldie" when she herself was in her 60s, and she often used it in reference to people who were much younger than herself. She's always pointing out oldies doing such things as driving about 40 miles per hour in the fast lane of the freeway or unconsciously and inconsiderately blocking supermarket aisles with their shopping carts.

One of her favorite oldie experiences occurred back when we were running the SugarFree Center. June answered the phone one day. It was a woman calling to cancel her appointment to learn how to use a meter. The reason she gave for canceling was, "You see, I'm 60 years old." June, who was 64 at the time, mused to herself, "What does being 60 have to do with canceling an appointment? . . . Oh well, I guess she's just an oldie."

When pressed to sum up exactly what an oldie is, June says it's a person who has given up on himself or herself. As we said before, that can happen at any age. But it's true that the older you grow the more temptation there is to fall victim to the oldie syndrome.

If you want to see whether you are developing incipient "oldieism," try taking the following test.

1. Do you use your age as an excuse for getting out of doing things?

2. Do you expect others to do special things for you? That is to say, do you have an "I need to be taken care of " turn of mind?

3. Even if you're financially well off and secure, do you feel poor and hesitate to spend money on yourself for things that would make you healthier and happier?

4. Do you use your age as an excuse—even if it's just to yourself—for being unhappy?

5. Do you generally resist trying new things?

6. Do you usually try to avoid responsibility?

7. If you're not retired yet, do you look forward to retirement as a time when you can "just do nothing"? If you *are* retired, do you spend most of your time "just doing nothing"?

8. Do you feel the best part of your life is over?

9. Do you focus on what you can't do rather than on what you can do?

10. Do you feel you're too old and that your mind doesn't work well enough now to try to work new electronic or technological devices—for example, the automatic teller machine at the bank, a computer, a VCR, or, most significantly, a blood sugar meter?

11. Do you often feel sorry for yourself?

12. Do you think more about the past than about the present and future?

13. Do you have a lot of regrets?

14. Do you have more things that you dread than things that you look forward to?

15. Do you often find yourself saying—or even thinking—such phrases as "What's the use?" or "It's just not worth the effort"?

16. Do you feel that you're too old to do most of the things you'd really like to do?

17. Do you primarily think of yourself and *your* needs rather than others and *their* needs?

Count how many yes answers you have. As you may have suspected, this quiz is like one of those "Are you an alcoholic?" quizzes in which even one yes answer is cause for concern. If you answered yes to one or more questions, you either are an oldie or are well on the way to becoming one.

But all is not lost. You don't have to be an oldie. Diabetes may be just the wake-up call you need to push you off the oldie track. We both practice oldie prevention with every fiber of our beings and it must be working at least a little. A few years ago after a talk we gave in Salt Lake City, a woman came up to us and said, "I hope you'll take this in the right way, but from reading your books, I'd think you're a lot younger than you really are." We did take it in the right way—except she was a little wrong in her assessment. Our real ages are not necessarily the ones that our birth certificates would indicate—and neither is yours. We recently heard a saying attributed to the baseball player/philosopher Satchel Paige: "How old would you be if you didn't know how old you were?" Ponder that one a minute. And then possibly experience a little shudder of horror at the possibility that if you didn't know how old you were, you might be a decade or two older from the way you're conducting your life.

A famous yachtsman once said, "Somewhere in the corner of your heart, you're always 22 years old." Now's the time to find that corner and expand it until it occupies your whole heart. Because it still is possible for you to be 22 years old in all the ways that really count, and one of the most important of those ways is feeling that many wonderful moments lie ahead for you and starting to take good care of yourself so you can enjoy them to the fullest.

At your age—whatever that age may be—it *is* worth the bother and, more important, *you're* worth the bother.

—*June and Barbara*

A PAIR OF FOND FAREWELLS

One of the rules for giving a speech is, "Tell them what you're going to tell them. Tell them. Then tell them what you told them." The same rule holds true for a book. We've done the first two and now we'll end by each of us telling you the most important parts of what we already told you.

The first recap is written in the form of a rap song to help it stick in your mind. You might chant this to yourself when you're out on brisk walks.

The second is a loving valentine from Virginia: *"The Fifteen Commandments for Living Well with Diabetes."* (This means that it's 50 percent more difficult to have diabetes than to be a Christian!) As former librarians, it's hard for us to recommend the mutilation of a book, but we think you might like to cut this list out—unless this is a library book—and put it on your refrigerator or bathroom mirror or some other place where you'll see it frequently.

Diabetes Rap Wrap-up
by
Type II Live Crew
AKA June and Barbara

For II-D's

If, when you're diagnosed, you're thin,
The odds are you'll need insulin.

In fact, when all is said and done,
Your therapy is like Type I.

But cherish this one consolation:
You're much less prone to complications.

For II-R's

The pounds melt off before your eyes,
When you eat less fat and exercise.

Good control, what gives you that?
More exercise and much less fat.

Look great, feel great, you know you can
With an exercise-and-low-fat plan.

Another tip—you ought to try it—
Add heaps of fiber to your diet.

But above all else, remember please
This one Great Truth of your disease:

A pair of genes caused what you've got;
A character flaw YOU HAVE NOT!

THE DIABETES GOSPEL ACCORDING
TO VIRGINIA VALENTINE

Virginia's
Fifteen Commandments
for Living Well with Diabetes

1. Thou shalt find a doctor and diabetes educator who understand that Type II diabetes is not a character flaw and who will work with thee to achieve normal range blood sugar goals, and thou shalt honor them.

2. Thou shalt visit thy doctor and diabetes educator every three months for monitoring of thy diabetes with glycohemoglobin and checking for possible complications.

3. Thou shalt work with the dietitian to design a livable yet healthy diet (high fiber, low fat, low protein, low sugar, low salt) that includes goodies now and then so thou won't covet gooey sweets and pig out.

4. Thou shalt have thy blood pressure and cholesterol and triglycerides monitored every three months and follow the diet and medication regimen to get them in the normal range. Also ask thy doctor if thou should be taking a baby aspirin every day to lower thy risk of heart attack.

5. Thou shalt have thy urine checked for microalbuminuria (microscopic levels of protein) every year after five years of diabetes and have any urinary tract or bladder infections treated immediately.

6. Thou shalt see thy ophthalmologist at least annually.

7. Thou shalt care for thy teeth and gums daily and see thy dentist and hygienist every six months.

8. Thou shalt monitor thy blood glucose levels on a regular basis and especially do a test when thou does not want to.

9. Thou shalt check thy feet daily and see a podiatrist every two to three months.

10. Thou shalt wear thy medical ID tag now and forever.

11. Thou shalt not smoke nor take up any tobacco products.

12. Thou shalt get a flu shot every year and thou shalt wear thy seat belt at all times whither thou goest.

13. If thou art woman and thy womb be fertile, thou shalt remember that bad blood sugars beget big bad babies with health problems. Do not beget any babies until thy blood sugars art in perfect control and thy doctor hath blessed any begettin'.

14. Thou shalt do something every day in the way of a healthy and pleasurable activity for thy body, thy mind, and thy spirit.

15. Thou shalt love thyself as a worthwhile person with many wonderful qualities and facets and not flog thyself for having diabetes or for the occasional blooper blood glucose.

AMEN